An indispensable boo~~~~~~~~~~~~~rson who feels
concerned for his own ~~~~~~~~~~~~~~~s.

DR~~~~~
VISION TRAINING
PROGRAMME

[Eye-care and vision-care for everyone]

by

Dr. Dhiren Gala
B.Sc., D.H.M.S., D.O., D.Ac.,
C.G.O., C.C.H., A.R.S.H.

Recipient of a gold medal for extraordinary
work in the field of Alternative Therapeutics

With

Dr. D. R. Gala
N.D., D.N.O., D.C.O.

Dr. Sanjay Gala
M.B. (BOM.), M.S. (ENT)

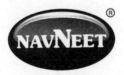

NAVNEET PUBLICATIONS (INDIA) LIMITED

Navneet House, Gurukul Road,	**Navneet Bhavan,** B. S. Road,
Memnagar, Ahmadabad – 380 052.	Dadar, Mumbai – 400 028.
Phone : 6630 5000	Phone : 6662 6565

DHANLAL BROTHERS DISTRIBUTORS
70, Princess Street, Mumbai – 400 002.
Phone : 2201 7027 / 2205 3716

G 4511

Visit us at : www.navneet.com | e-mail : npil@navneet

Dr. Dhiren Gala
1st Floor, Abbas Building 'A',
Near Tilak Market, Jalbhai Lane,
Harkishandas Hospital Road,
Grant Road (East), Mumbai – 400 004.
Phone : 2386 7275

Timings : 4.00 to 7.00 p.m.

PREFACE

It is our belief that as patients we are too passive about our health and well-being. With scant and sometimes incorrect information, we are often not able to make intelligent choices about the protection and enhancement of our vision. The attitude in the past has been to leave the development of vision and eyes to change. But we maintain that because of the demands our technological culture places on vision, 'development by change' will no longer suffice. We cannot alter the society or the situation; We can foster such eyes and vision as would meet the needs of the time. We can improve on our 'stone age' eyes.

With this in mind, we are providing information from a wide variety of field : optometry, nutrition, child development, psychology and physiology. All of these are related to our visual sense. We are sure that this information will enable the reader to take the right steps to protect not only his or her own vision but also that of the generations to come.

Many of us suffer from some degree of vision impairment— inefficiencies, fatigue, discomfort, strain, near-sightedness, farsightedness or minor muscular imbalances. Many a time, we remain unaware of the fact that the trouble stems from our eyes and end up at a doctor's dispensary complaining of aches and pains. Undue tiredness, lethargy, mental tension, easy irritability, anger, rigidity – all these can be symptoms or results of visual problems. Inefficiency of eyes can go a long way in playing havoc with our moods and bodies. Even when aware of the visual problems, we often feel resigned to them. At the most, we put on glasses, ignoring the real sources of our problems. As a result, vision grows worse over the years and glasses grow stronger and thicket.

However, we need not watch helplessly such deterioration of vision. We can greatly improve the efficiency of eyes and the quality of vision through 'vision therapy'.

Some time back, a young man, who had failed the vision test required to become a pilot, came to us. It was his life's dream to fly, and he was disappointed and discouraged. Although he believed that he was condemned to spend his life on the ground, he came to see us. Very wary of trying and failing again, he approached the vision training programme sceptically. But within a month, scepticism had given way to enthusiasm. He passed the next vision test with 'flying' colours. To he is a happy pilot. In fact, every person who undertakes vision therapy experiences enhancement in the acuteness as well as the quality of vision.

We sincerely hope that this book will prove a stepping stone to a lifetime of strong eyes and healthy vision.

– Authors

CONTENTS

1. INTRODUCTION

Eyes are invaluable. Philosophers have called them windows to the soul. Yet they are probably the most neglected of all organs. The testimony to this is the fact that almost fifty per cent of our population wear glasses. An author has mentioned in a lighter vein that, 'If eligible young men choose to sidetrack bespectacled girls, their pickings are slim indeed !' The statement may seem a bit exaggerated, but it is nevertheless true. Visual problems are propping up at an alarming pace.

Only 2 to 3 per cent of the population have eye-problems at birth; yet possibly a full 70 per cent run into some kind of trouble with eyesight during their lifetimes. Statistics show that we are becoming a generation of visually handicapped. Nearsightedness, astigmatism and a variety of hidden visual problems such as co-ordination and perceptual difficulties related to eye-inefficiencies are all on the rise.

More often than not, we remain unaware of the problem. Since most eye examinations do not check for these hidden problems, they go undetected and consequently untreated. They include erratic eye-tracking, sluggish or inefficient focusing, unstable fusion (eye-teaming skills), reduced peripheral awareness, inadequate depth perception and awkward eye-to-body or eye-to-hand co-ordination. Persons suffering from such defects may experience trouble tracking a line across a page, shifting focus from far to near (or vice versa), difficulty in converging on an object or judging the distance and position of an object correctly. Some persons do not use both eyes together but one at a time.

Impaired visual skills narrow our field of vision and limit our perspective, sometimes leaving in their wake bizarre symptoms which seemingly have nothing to do with eyes or sight. Undue fatigue, easy irritability, mental tension, a stiff neck or an aching back, all could be symptoms of a visual defect.

5

Had we still been living free in the wilds, our eyes probably would not have run into the kinds of trouble they do today when we require them to take on tasks for which they are not biologically prepared. It is like asking someone who has never run a mile to compete for the marathon in the Olympics. Our eyes valiantly try to go the distance but may fade in the stretch and breakdown. It does not always put us in eyeglasses or become as obvious as a crossed eye; but it does cause confusion at the subconscious level and often leads to those vague aches and pains or fatigue at the end of the day which drags us to the bed as soon as we walk in doors. Those who listen to their bodies will quit before the spine is permanently curved or the burning in the stomach has been converted into an ulcer or the migraine has come to stay; but not all listen well, or at all. The attitude of this society is to prize the mighty intellect and to reward the indefatigable student.

What are we doing to ourselves to impair our vision and wear out our eyes while the rest of our body remains strong? You are doing it right at this minute as you concentrate on little black marks on a page which you translate into meaning. Now there is not much wrong with that; it is doing it hour after hour without respite that is harmful. The problem is that we have left-over eyes. They evolved during the ages to work well for the hunter and the country farmer, but they are not suited for the life we lead today. A city-dweller uses his eyes in vastly different ways than did the man who hunted and gathered fruits or edible roots all day long. Today we rely upon our eyes for between 80 to 90 per cent of the information we receive about the world. Our eyes have always done their best to accommodate us; but they cannot change overnight – or in a century.

Though looking at distance is natural and restful for the eyes, we barely give them a chance to do so. In fact, we continuously engage them in near-point work, concentrating on minute details.

During his school years, an average student ploughs through some 150 books, i.e., 15 books a year. In college, the number jumps to anywhere from 20 to 30. This gives little time for the eyes to do what they do best : look towards the horizon.

Even after completing studies, there is no respite for the poor eyes. A doctor will have to make time at night to plough through medical journals if he is going to stay abreast of what's happening in his field; an engineer or an architect will continue to draw plans; an accountant will remain busy with numbers; a fabric designer will spend her days working on intricate patterns.

What has happened is that the amount of work we are asking of our eyes is greater than what they are made to handle. And like an overworked radiator in a car caught in stop-and-go traffic, they break down. Glasses have become the badges of courage handed to persons who choose to push through the massive amount of material society expects them to digest.

Now several things occur when we ask the mind to be alert and think critically : our muscles tense and our breathing becomes shallow. We adapt our whole body into a 'Fighting' posture 'The book may be difficult but I will get through it,' we consciously or unconsciously tell ourselves.

And later, when we end up with a sore back, we do not feel like going for an outing or playing a badminton match. In effect the eyes and the body say : 'Are you crazy ? We are tired and stiff and want some time off.....' And we end up or relax by watching television or reading a magazine article on how to plant a money-plant in a window box ! The material is not as difficult, but we are still looking at little marks on a page or just sitting motionless.

In short, we engage our eyes the whole day long in tasks for which they are not yet evolutionally ready. Incorrect and excessive use of the eyes and inadequate rest to the eyes are the chief causes of visual problems. Add faulty nutrition and inflexible visual style and the list is complete.

We have been made to understand that most eye defects are hereditory and, therefore, largely unchangeable. Therefore, we have come to accept the idea that there is basically nothing we can do to change the situation except wear glasses. To the contrary, abundant research indicates it is unlikely that the breakdown is programmed into the species; there is solid evidence that we are doing something to cause it.

If visual problems are of our doing, we can take steps to undo them. That is what VISION THERAPY is all about.

We need such eyes as would allow us to perform a wide spectrum of tasks—near as well as distant—with equal ease. And developing such eyes is a comparatively easy task. The succeeding pages will enlighten you about how to accomplish this goal.

2. WHAT IS VISION THERAPY ?

"Do you understand ?" he asked.

"Yes, I see." she replied.

Such overlapping of meaning in language is not simply an accident. It undoubtedly is the result of early man's perception that vision and comprehension are intimately linked. But as science attempted to explain eyesight by comparing the eye with a camera, the concept that 'sight is related to insight' got lost in the new technology that permeated our thinking. The time has come to revise this attitude, for now we can explain and put into practice an idea which has been around since times immemorial : Vision is not only what we see, but also what we are prepared to perceive.

Vision is much more than opening the eyes, the way one might turn on a television set. The ability to comprehend what we see is a process involving the brain as well as the eyes. It has developed through trial and error. The way Homo sapiens sees today is the result of his development through the ages; the way each individual sees is the product of his or her own development throughout his or her lifetime.

Vision is an active process which begins at birth and constantly undergoes minor shifts and alterations due to : (1) a basic predisposition to a specific personality, evident at birth, (2) biochemical influences or nutrition and (3) the physical environment.

To put it in other words, vision is no mere passive occurrence like breathing, but is, instead, a complex and learned process which occurs mainly in the brain. The way we think affects our vision and our vision affects the way we think. Impaired visual skills narrow our field of vision and limit our perspective. By improving our visual skills, much as we can improve co-ordination of other parts of the body, we can realise an expanded perspective or vision.

Good vision is much more than acuity, which only refers to how clearly you can see. It involves a whole spectrum of skills, viz., How well can you use both eyes together ? How quickly can you judge left from right ? How well do you see objects in space ? Can you shift focus from near to far (or vice versa) quickly and easily ? How good is your visual memory ? Are your visual skills equal to your age or needs ? Besides, vision is tied up with how you move, think or come to a decision. In fact, your visual problems provide a clue to what kind of stresses you operate under. Distortions of eyes are considered to be problems in reaching a decision, reflections of behavioural style and indications of some form of stress, whether it be psychological or environmental.

Yet at the present time, most routine eye-examinations just check for disease and test visual acuity on a chart that is well over hundred years old. You may do remarkably well reading those small letters and be disease-free, but you can still be walking around with a load of hidden visual problems which can do anything from making you rigid or cranky in your outlook, giving you a backache or making you seem less intelligent than you are. You may know you have got good ideas in your head, but you just don't seem to get them out. And the block in the passageway could be an inefficient visual system.

The basic premise of vision therapy is that vision is learned. Since that is so, we can learn to see properly – if we have been doing anything wrong – with proper guidance. Vision therapy is a method to train the entire visual system including the brain to operate at peak efficiency.

Vision therapy includes a series of exercises and behaviour modification drills which will help an individual unlearn many incorrect visual responses or habits. It is a means of helping a person develop healthy vision, undistorted and flexible enough to meet all possible needs, right from reading a book to spot a horse on the horizon.

The traditional approach to visual problems has so far been to prescribe glasses and do no more. The real causes of visual disturbances are not sought. Vision therapy, however, strikes at the root of the problem. It begins with the premise that vision can be protected from deteriorating, developed to its full potential and enhanced to meet any special need. Vision therapy can help prevent, control or even diminish nearsightedness or farsightedness.

Following vision therapy, behaviour or personality, too, may change for the better. However, changes in behaviour are always more subtle than the visual changes. A person in whom a particular way of acting and reacting has been ingrained for decades cannot be expected to wake up one morning and find that the old patterns have dissipated with dreams.

Vision therapy is divided into three parts : (1) Assessment of visual style and present visual status, (2) Exercising and (3) Maintenance. These parts work together to bring about favourable changes in our visual habits and teach us the correct use of the eyes.

(1) **Assessment** : Most of us take vision for granted. We are not aware of how we use (or abuse) our eyes. We do not know what the results of our visual habits are. Assessment involves learning to identify our visual style and personality and pinpointing our specific visual problems, such as near-sightedness (myopia), farsightedness (hypermetropia), astigmatism, lazy eye or muscular imbalances.

Our visual style is the way we use our eyes to collect visual information. Even in the smallest of daily tasks, we make choices about what we focus our eyes on and what we ignore. We may love reading or have a fascination for what is going on around us. We may hate puzzles but love driving, be fascinated by architectural details or vast panoramas. Whatever catches our eyes affects their development. Our lenses and muscles become programmed to work in set patterns. Year after year, we repeat these patterns, these visual habits. This can lead to unnecessary eye-strain or limit our flexibility in gathering visual perceptions. An inflexible style may worsen existing visual defects.

Self-assessment helps us to become aware of these daily habits. Through a series of tests, we become conscious of our visual style. A detailed questionnaire helps us to realise how we use and apply our visual style in various daily situations.

We then combine this information with the results of specific tests that reveal the presence or absence of nearsightedness, farsightedness, astigmatism, lazy eye, fusion problems or other muscular imbalances. We learn to recognise how our eyes feel when we focus or relax them.

This process of self-assessment works hand-in-hand with our eye-doctor's continuing care. It is undesirable to practise any therapy solely on one's own. However, informed self-care when combined with professional attention, provides a solid base for improvement of vision.

(2) **Exercising** : After the process of assessment and self-assessment, we can select the training programme that will work on our particular vision problems. The exercise programmes are designed to concentrate on the management of nearsightedness or farsightedness. They can be combined with special supplementary programmes that stress exercises for lazy eye, suppression, inadequate fusion or muscular imbalances.

Each programme consists of a four-week series of daily exercises. One half-hour a day is all the time that is needed. Each exercise is followed by a weekly evaluation section so that we can measure our progress. We see our range of clear vision increase, find that we do not have to depend on our glasses so much, happily observe the eye-strain diminishing and become more flexible in our visual style.

These exercises are effective because the inner working of the eye can be favourably influenced. We can change the way we focus and fix our gaze. Those of us who are nearsighted need to release focus; those of us who are farsighted need to increase it. This can be accomplished through exercises involving simple techniques.

Though the programmes require commitment and sincerity, they are not complicated. In fact, the exercises are easy and provide fun.

When performing the exercises remember these tips :

(1) Read through each exercise before beginning. Get familiar with it. Understand its purpose and goals.

(2) Perform the exercises in a well illuminated, quiet place. Sit on a comfortable chair or stand erect with weight evenly balanced.

(3) Do not overdo the exercises. Keep the focus soft. Let the body and eyes be relaxed. Vision improves from relaxation and not from eye-strain.

(4) Do not expect instant results. Build visual strength slowly. The programmes lead, step by step, to better vision.

Do not skip an exercise or rush. It is necessary to repeat an exercise over and over again to gain mastery over it.

(5) Learn to identify personal visual style in all daily activities. Be on the lookout for incorrect outlook.

(6) Practise those exercises that seem difficult again and again. Challenge yourself.

(3) Maintenance : Once we have improved our vision, we would like to maintain it that way. Therefore, we must continue doing the exercises at least once a week. If we feel that our vision is deteriorating, we can repeat the four-week programme.

The two most important parts of maintenance are : (1) Keeping a high level of self-awareness about how we use our eyes and (2) Spending time without glasses as often as possible.

Once we are aware of the ways we abuse our eyes through the bad visual habits that we have developed, we must be on our guard. We do not want to slip back into old, destructive patterns.

Whenever we are doing activities that do not require clear and sharp vision, we should take off our glasses. The progressive development or worsening of eye problems can be slowed down or halted altogether by this simple technique. Unless glasses are periodically taken off, the eyes cannot attain their full potential.

In conclusion, it can be said that vision therapy is a system which helps us change our approach to visual perception. We learn to recognise our visual style. We become aware of the way we use our eyes to view the world.

Vision training also teaches us how to use the physical components of our eyes. We learn about the crystalline lens and various eye muscles and their functions. We learn to change the way we focus and move our eyes.

This dual approach helps us overcome incorrect mental and physical habits that lower natural visual acuity.

Although some people who undergo training may end up no longer needing glasses, and indeed this may be the reason you picked up this book, the aim of vision therapy is much more than that. Vision therapy offers a means of protecting and enhancing your own vision and that of the next generations. Vision therapy is an experience in perception. Its aim : seeing everything !

-----

3. THE EYE AND THE VISION

The structure of the eye : The eye is one of the most important organs and probably the most useful of various sense organs of our body. No wonder, nature has protected

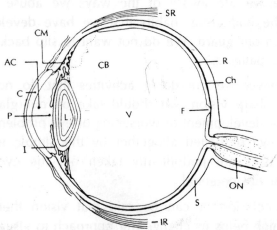

C – cornea	S – sclera	Ch – choroid
R – retina	AC – aqueous chamber	I – iris
P – pupil	CM – ciliary muscle	CB – ciliary body
V – vitreous	F – fovea	ON – optic nerve
SR – superior rectus	IR – inferior rectus	
muscle	muscle	

Fig. 3.1

the eyes by lodging them into conical bony sockets called orbits.

Only about 1/6th of the eyeball is externally visible. This part, too, is protected by the eyelids.

The eyeball is made up of three concentric coats : (1) the outer, fibrous sclera (also called the white of the eye), (2) the middle blood-vascular choroid and (3) the inner, nervous retina.

The sclera is thick, tough, white and opaque. It maintains the shape of the eye, protects the inner structures and creates darkness inside the eye.

The centre of the front part of the eye has a thin, transparent watchglass-like coat called cornea. The rays of light coming from various objects are bent by the cornea to bring them to a focus on the retina.

The middle coat of the eye, i.e., the choroid is made up chiefly of blood-vessels and hence nourishes the eye.

The inner retina consists of numerous nerve cells which receive light rays coming from the outside world, convert them into electrical impulses and transmit them to the brain.

The black or darkbrown (sometimes yellowish, bluish or greenish) part of the eye, is called the iris. It lies exactly behind the cornea. At the centre of the iris is a small circular opening called the pupil, which allows the light rays to enter the eye and controls their intensity by changing its own size (i.e., the pupil contracts in bright light and expands in dim light).

Behind the iris is the crystalline lens, which is normally transparent. It is held in place by 72 suspensory ligaments. When this lens becomes opaque, the person is said to be suffering from cataract.

From the back of the eyeball starts the optic nerve which conveys the electrical impulses originating in the retina to the brain.

That part of the brain which is concerned with vision is called the visual cortex. It is here that the impulses coming from the retina are processed and interpreted and the person 'sees'.

The harmonious and co-ordinated movements of the two eyes are brought about by six pairs of muscles, four of which are called the 'recti muscles' and two are called the 'obliqui muscles'.

The function of the eye : The main function of the eye is obviously : seeing. Our eye is a wonderfully efficient organ. It produces images by collecting and processing the reflected rays of light that bounce off the surface of everything around us. As soon as the light touches our eyes, the pupil responds, contracting or dilating. Once it passes through the pupil, the light is directed by the lens to the image transmission centre of the eye, i.e., the retina. The retina transforms the light images into encoded electrical impulses that travel to the brain, where they are registered, evaluated and reacted to in an instant.

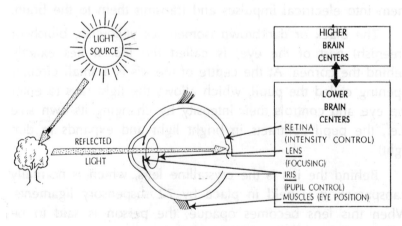

Fig. 3.2

Thus, the eyes are only 'light collecting' centres; actual seeing is the function of the brain. The information gathered by eyes is combined within the brain with our knowledge, memory and emotions. Vision is the product of this blend. That is why visual training is also concerned with behaviour and visual style. What we see in our mind's eye, how our personality views the world, is as important as how our eyeballs collect light.

Binocular vision : We have to consider the fact that we have two eyes, each looking at the world from a slightly different angle or perspective. Though each eye forms its own image, we don't see double because the two images are 'fused' by the brain to give rise to a single, three-dimensional, properly located picture.

There are two requisites for fusion : (1) The light entering the two eyes, as they look at the same object, must fall on corresponding points on the two retinae and (2) the two images formed on the two retinae must be almost equally clear. If these two conditions are not met, fusion may develop only partially or not at all.

Loss of fusion :

(1) Due to unequal clarity of images formed on the two retinae : As said above, the images transmitted from the two eyes must be almost equally clear for full fusion to occur. If this is not the case, the brain is receiving an image from one eye that is far less clear than that from the other. The brain cannot combine these two dissimilar pictures without lowering the clarity of sight that is achieved by the stronger eye alone. Therefore, the brain automatically turns off the weaker eye's picture. This causes a variety of vision problems; but it serves to allow the clearest possible sight from the stronger eye.

(2) Due to misalignment of the eyes : If both the eyes are not directed at the object we are viewing (as happens in squint), non-corresponding areas of the two retinae are stimulated and the brain receives two non-fusable images. The brain then selects the one image that is clear and correctly located and ignores the other image to prevent double vision.

Such turning off or ignoring the image, on the part of brain, is termed 'suppression'. If suppression is detected before it becomes an entrenched neurological response, it is easy to eliminate it by strengthening specific eye muscles and promoting the vision of the weak eye.

However, if suppression goes on for too long, it can lead to more serious vision problems. The neural connections between the suppressed eye and the brain suffer from disuse and even glasses cannot 'wake up' the weak eye to its full potential. Such eye is termed 'lazy' or 'amblyopic' eye.

If amblyopia (or laziness of the eye) is caught early, it can often be corrected by exercises. If long-standing amblyopia cannot be fully corrected, vision training exercises must also be directed at the 'strong' eye to relieve it of undue strain and prevent development of a fresh refractive error of worsening of an existing one. A large number of children who have a lazy eye, develop nearsightedness in their strong, working eye unless they perform exercises to improve the binocular balance.

4. HOW TO USE THE EYES ?

Faulty ways of using the eyes are sources of eye-strain and lead to the development of visual defects. If you wish to care for your own eyes and those of your children, you should know and learn the correct ways of using the eyes. The correct use of the eyes will, more or less, ensure the maintenance of good vision, reduce the chances of the development of new visual defects and prevent further deterioration of existing visual defects.

Reading and writing : As has been stated at numerous places earlier, our eyes are meant to look at distance. Near works such as reading, writing etc. are, so to say, unnatural for our eyes. But these are the very tasks that society prizes. We cannot avoid all the close-range or near-point work that is required today; however, we can make life a little easier for our eyes by following certain simple rules.

(1) Always read or write in the sitting position, i.e., you should be seated at a desk in a comfortable chair (not on the floor), not lying on your stomach or on your side. Keep your head and the back straight, and not tilted to any side. Do not stoop forward.

The desk or table should be at waist level when you are seated. Working at a surface too high gives as much distortion as viewing a movie from the front row. The chair should be such as would permit the feet to remain planted on the floor; if the feet do not touch the floor, use a small stool or phone-books or a box under them.

(2) The illumination of the book should also be consi-dered. It is necessary that the place where you read or write is very well lighted. If reading during the day in natural daylight, preferably sit near a window in such a way that the shadow of the hand does not fall on the book. If reading at night, position the lamp such that the light comes from your left (presuming that you are a right-hander). The lamp should be good enough to provide strong illumination.

(3) It is desirable that the book you read has nonglossy paper, reasonably big types (letters) and good printing.

(4) The material you read should be in front of your eyes and at a distance at least equal to the length between your knuckles and elbows. In simple terms, hold the material in front of you so that your elbow makes a right angle when you are holding the book.

(5) The inclination of the book is also important. The text should be parallel to the plane of your face, not flat on the desk, which is why desks constructed at a 20-degree incline are better for reading and writing than horizontal surfaces.

The parents of a scholar – or anyone who reads and writes a great deal – should consider constructing a simple inclined platform to set on a desk. Such an inclined desk enables a person to read more efficiently with less effort on the part of eyes. Flat surfaces cause the visual system to work harder to make up for the distortion.

If you choose to hold the book you are reading in your hands, hold it up so that the pages are parallel to the plane of your face. Do not allow the book to lie on your lap.

(6) Blink more often when you are reading or writing. Quite some persons forget to blink when they are engrossed in reading. One blink per line is the minimum requirement. Initially, this blinking may have to be done consciously. Later on, however, it becomes a habit. Staring contributes to eye-strain and blinking provides rest to the eyes.

(7) Do not block out peripheral vision, which is a common practice of people who get too involved in close, detailed work. Try not to be distracted, but be aware of what is going on around you.

(8) While reading or writing, make sure that you are breathing properly. If your breathing is shallow, take a few deep breaths now and then.

(9) Perhaps the single most important factor in protecting your eyes when you read is to take a break approximately every 20 minutes. For the average reader, this means taking a break after every 3-4 pages of non-fiction reading or every 8-10 pages of fiction reading. Look up across the room or out of the window, at distant objects. Continue to do so for at least two minutes. Do not resume near-point work till the distant objects are quite clear. It may seem a waste of time to look out of the window every so often. But in the end, you may not get as tired as you would otherwise be; you may be able to absorb more; the most important point is that you won't push your eyes past the point where there is nothing they can do except adapt to the strain they are under and so give you trouble when you want to do something else–like see clearly at a hundred feet or play cricket.

(10) After an hour of reading or writing, get up and stretch. Move around. Take deep breaths. Look at the horizon. Ensure that your distant vision is as clear as it was before you sat down to read.

(11) Do not indulge in close-range work, by keeping awake till late hours. Remember that your eyes need more rest than your body.

(12) Never read in a moving vehicle. Similarly, do not read when you are sick. Reading may keep you from being bored while you are travelling or bedridden. But surely, you won't like to drive away boredom at the cost of good sight.

Television : Although the television manufacturers assure us that radiation leakage (X-rays) has been reduced to little or none as long as the set is in good working order, you might as well take the precaution of sitting at least five or six feet away from the screen. This is particularly important if you own a colour television. Albeit, do not sit so far away that you have to strain your eyes to see details.

Never watch television in a darkened room, even if it is a late night movie. The illumination of the room should ideally be such as would match that of the television screen. In any case, keep a small light on.

While watching television, sit comfortably, with the back fully supported and the head drooping slightly backward so that the eyes remain partly shut. Take a break every now and then, just as suggested while doing close-range work.

Sewing, knitting etc. : Sewing and knitting are also close-range jobs and suggestions made while discussing 'reading' are applicable here too.

Do not stare at the cloth or the stitches. Keep the eyesight moving along with the needle or the pin.

5. HOW TO REST THE EYES ?

Excessive use of and inadequate rest to the eyes is one of the causes of most visual problems. Very few persons know how to rest the eyes effectively. Given below are some simple measures which bring about profound relief and provide relaxation to the eyes. Any one or more of these measures can be employed to rest tired and gritty eyes.

(1) Palming : This is a method par excellence to remove eye-fatigue.

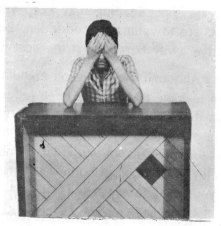

Fig. 5.1

Sit on a chair, with a desk in the front. Close the eyes and lightly cover them with palms (with the finger crossing at right angles), as shown in the figure. Place the palms in such a way that the nose remains uncovered and the eyes remain behind the slight hollows of the palms. Rest the elbows on the desk. The aim is to prevent light rays from reaching or entering the eyes. Hence take care to leave no gaps between the fingers or between the edge of the palms and the nose.

Take deep breaths. Think of some happy incident; or visualise a distant scene. Continue to do so for 2 to 3 minutes or more.

(2) **Looking at distant objects :** As stated at a number of places in this book, our eyes are made to look at distance. Just looking at distant objects rests the eyes. If the eyes feel stiff or tired following prolonged work at close-range (e.g., reading, writing, watching television etc.), they can be rested by looking at the horizon for a few minutes.

(3) **Rythmic movements :** Leisurely and gentle rythmic movements bring about muscle-relaxation and alleviate strain. A variety of rythmic movements can be undertaken to relax the muscles of the eyes and the body.

(a) Bar swings :

Stand in front of a window or a door which has verticle bars or grill. Through the bars, direct your gaze to distant objects. Now sway slowly and rythmically, like the pendulum of a clock. Transfer your weight from one foot to the other. Keep the body muscles limp and lax. Breathe rythmically. Continue to do so for 2 to 3 minutes or more.

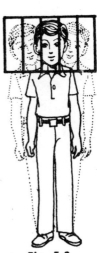

Fig. 5.2

(b) Round swings :

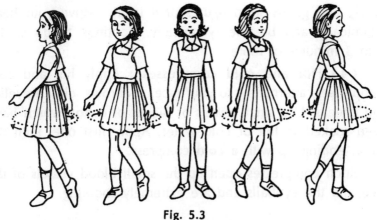

Fig. 5.3

Stand keeping a distance of 8 to 10 inches between the two feet. With the help of the left forefoot, slowly turn to your right, through 90 degrees. Let the arms swing along with your body. Revert to the original position. Now without stopping and with the help of the right forefoot, slowly turn to your left, through 90 degrees. Let the arms swing along with your body. Throughout the procedure, breathe rythmically and direct your gaze to low-lying distant objects. Continue this motion for 2 to 3 minutes or more.

(c) Head movements :

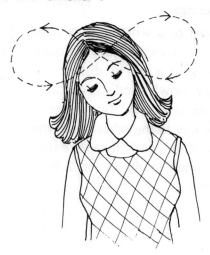

Fig. 5.4

Sit comfortably. Keep the eyes closed. With your head, slowly and gently form figures of 8 in air. Move your head rythmically and breathe rythmically. Continue to do so for 2 to 3 minutes of more.

(4) **Hot and cold compresses :** Apply hot and cold compresses, alternately, to your face, eyebrows, closed eyelids and cheeks. Use small towels or pieces of cotton which have been soaked in hot or cold water. Apply first one, then the other, ending up with a cold compress.

Such compresses open up the small blood vessels of the face and the eyeballs and are extremely soothing.

(5) Water splashes : For a few seconds, sprinkle cold water from a running tap, on the closed eyes. Thereafter, do not wipe the water on the face with a towel; allow it to dry on its own.

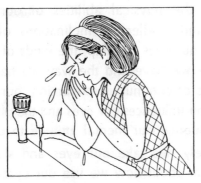

Fig. 5.5

(6) Massage of the face and the eyes : With the help of a napkin soaked in warm (or hot) water, vigorously rub the skin of the forehead, cheeks and the neck. However, the eyes should not be rubbed.

Follow this up by gently massaging the forehead and the closed eyelids with the finger-tips.

This will relieve the tension in facial and eye muscles.

(7) Magnet Therapy* : Magnetic treatment, too, has been found to be immensely useful in bringing about relaxation of the eye-muscles. Special magnetic frames are available, which can be worn on the face for 5 to 10 minutes. Cool magnetic waves emanating from the magnets rest the eyes and relieve strain.

---

* Details about Magnet Therapy have been presented in chapter 14.

6. SELF-ASSESSMENT : PART ONE

As stated earlier, our visual style or the way we employ our eyes to collect information has a definite bearing upon our visual status. Each of us has his own visual style. It is our personal way of using our eyes to view the world. It evolves as a result of the physical abilities of our eyes and the psychological and intellectual inclinations of our minds. It affects the way our eyes develop, the kinds of visual strengths and weeknesses we have and the way we handle perceptual tasks. In a cycle of continuous interaction, our mental attitude toward perception influences our eyes and the physical responses of our eyes influence our mental attitude to perception.

Unfortunately, we take our eyes and sight for granted. We seldom think about how we use our eyes. It is necessary to realise how we approach visual tasks so that we can identify potential visual problems, areas of visual stress and general perceptional handicaps. To gain self-awareness, we need to understand the connection between how we see and how we think.

There are two general categories of visual style : fixated-central and scanning-peripheral. Most of us use either of these two styles, depending upon the task on hand. However, we tend to fall into one category more than the other. Let us have a look at these basic styles and understand how they affect the working of our eyes.

FIXATED-CENTRAL STYLE

If we are comfortable with detail, enjoy reading and closed visual spaces, we are probably fixated-central. We direct our gaze to objects close to us. We are attracted to all print, read every word and rarely skim. Our eyes are converged or overconverged most of the time. We are probably nearsighted, or will be some day.

26

When combined with high endurance, the fixated-central visual style leads to a vision-intensive approach to perception. People with this style can usually concentrate and read for long periods of time.

The result of this style is that the crystalline lens is put in a bulged position most of the time. This may lead to lens inflexibility and produce sluggishness when shifting focus from near to far. The long-term result of high endurance, fixated-central visual style is worsening nearsightedness.

The high endurance, fixated-central style seems a blessing in our present culture. Despite problems of eye-strain, increasing nearsightedness and focal inflexibility, people who are able to concentrate on detail hour after hour and to handle close-range or near-point tasks are well suited to society's demands. Years of complex and competitive schooling and high esteem for well-read persons who do white-collar jobs make this style seem useful. Because of the acceptance and praise that fixated-central people receive, they often ignore (or are unaware of) the possible harmful side-effects of this style until it has begun to affect their vision.

Sometimes, however, fixated-central viewing may be combined with low endurance. Headaches, limited concentration and general visual discomfort are the results. If this is our style, we are trapped. Not inclined or able to use our eyes in a general scanning way, we are stuck with a focally intense style that causes problems. We cannot enjoy the pleasures of reading. The crystalline lens is constantly being strained by the impulse to focus on nearby objects. Muscle strain and fatigue make convergence hard to maintain. Endurance gets lower and lower. Headaches or even nervous tension can result.

Note : Vision and mind are intimately related. Specific visual habits or traits are often combined with certain mental attitudes and intellectual approaches. If we have a fixated-central visual style, we will tend to be well ordered and methodical in our pursuit of information. Children who possess this style may spend many hours reading alone. They are generally well organised and are good about finishing a task once it is begun. As adults, they tend to have good memories, are avid readers and are successful at work. If excessively fixated-central, they may have trouble integrating separate pieces of information into larger concepts for practical application.

In both types of fixated-central styles, appropriate eye-exercises, development of focal flexibility and use of relaxation techniques can lessen physical strain and resulting visual problems.

SCANNING-PERIPHERAL STYLE

If we enjoy visual tasks that require a general overview, like sports and outdoor activities (or occupations) and dislike close-range or near-point activities, we are probably scanning-peripheral. This style is usually corelated with farsightedness or no noticeable refractive (visual) error.

In general, this information collecting style is the way most children view the world. Farsighted at birth, they learn about their environment by constantly collecting impressions and information from all around them. They do not rely upon eyes alone for information collection. Touch, taste, smell, hearing—all are equally important. Since the crystalline lens is very flexible in young children, they are usually not troubled while performing close-range or near-point tasks.

Adults who retain a scanning-peripheral style may use their eyes to amass a lot of general information, to become aware of much that goes on around them. But they may be handicapped by the inability to handle close-range or near-point tasks. If they have a visually demanding job, they are likely to work slowly, to depend upon conversation or other clues to gain information. They may suffer from eye-strain and discomfort when forced to do prolonged close-range or near-point work.

The crystalline lens in the scanning-peripheral eye is flattened and often slow or unresponsive to the demand for lens-bulge (e.g., while reading). If the nature of work makes it necessary to do a lot of near-point work, eye-strain, headache or general fatigue may result.

> Note : A scanning-peripheral style can cause carelessness and a haphazard approach to learning and concentration. This style can limit the amount of reading we do, limit our ability to acquire new written information and increase our interest in T.V. and radio. Adults who possess this style can be quick-witted, given to theoretical thinking and comfortable with creative, self-generated ideas. However, they may be frustrated by the inability to collect and deal with detailed visual information at home and on the job.

There are advantages and disadvantages of either of these visual styles. Problems arise when we get locked into one style, i.e., cannot alter it even when necessary. If this happens, we cannot get the most out of whichever situation we find ourselves in. A balance between the two styles promotes visual acuity and physical as well as intellectual health.

The next part of this chapter contains a number of simple tests and questionnaires to detect our present personality and visual style. Parents should try to judge their children's personality and visual style. Once we have become aware of our visual style (and therefore its limitations), we can make conscious efforts to make it more balanced and thus eliminate possibilities of development or deterioration of visual errors in the future.

DETECTING VISUAL STYLE

(1) Visual approach

Apparatus   : Figure 6.1

Glasses   : Use glasses only if absolutely necessary to see the picture clearly.

Children   : Same routine as adults.

Routine   : Study the picture given below for three seconds (count three). Close the eyes and cover the picture. Then answer the questions that follow.

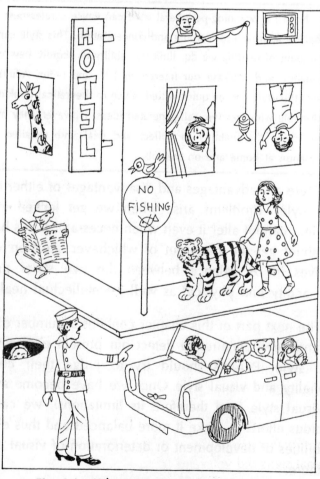

Fig. 6.1 : What's Wrong With This Picture ?

Describe the scene generally : ....

....

In the picture, there were how many persons ? ....
cars ? .... buildings ? .... printed signs ? ....
How many riders were there in the car ? ....
Was the building made of brick, wood or concrete ? ....
Did you see a pattern on any person's clothing ? What pattern
was it ? .... Did you read any sign ? What did it
say ? .... Did you notice anything unusual in
the picture ? .... Did you first notice the street, the
building or human figures ? ....

Now uncover the picture and glance at it for the count of
six. Cover the picture again. Answer the following questions :
What new parts of the picture did you see ? ....
What caught your eye this time ? ....
In the picture, there were how many persons ? ....
cars ? .... buildings ? .... printed signs ? ....
What did the printed signs say ? ....

....

Did you see anything unusual in the picture ? ....

....

Did the picture show trees ? .... the sun ? ....
.... the moon ? .... the sky ? .... List all
the objects you noticed in the picture ....

....

Uncover the picture again and look at it for the count of
ten. Answer the following questions :
What did you see that you had overlooked earlier ?.........

....

What signs did you read ? ....

Did you notice the television ? .... an umbrella ?
.... the manhole ? .... the policeman ?
.... the pig ? .... the white car ? ....
Did you see the man with a dog ? .... the man without arms ? .... the fish ?

Did you notice the man sitting backward in the car ? .... the policeman's jacket ? .... the misprinted signs ? .... List all the objects you noticed

....

....

....

Evaluation

On first viewing :

(1) Did you notice general shapes, outlines and textures ?..

(2) Did you notice a few objects in detail ? ....

(3) Did you notice large or small objects ? ....

(4) Did you read printed signs ? ....

(5) Did you catch any of the unusual features of the picture ? ....

On second viewing :

(1) Did you change your visual approach from general to particular or vice versa ? ....

(2) How much more detail did you pick up ? ....

(3) Did you read most of the signs ? ....

(4) Did you see most of the persons, animals or cars ? ....

(5) Did you catch more of the unusual features of the picture ? ....

On third viewing :

(1) What did you concentrate upon ? Minute details or general overview ? ....

(2) Did you feel you had seen the whole picture ?..........

(3) Are you still curious about the picture ? ....
Or are you bored ? ....

> **Note :** During the three-second and six-second stints, the most desirable and well-balanced response to this test is to register the basic 'theme' and overall contents of the picture while noticing some specific details. Persons with a fixated-central visual style find some difficulty in picking up the general theme of the picture but do identify details. On the other hand, persons with a peripheral-scanning visual style easily comprehend the general theme of the picture but pick up only a few details or have difficulty in remembering them.

(2) Visual style in everyday situations :

(A) Reading :

(1) How many hours a day do you spend reading ?
....

(2) What do you read ? Newspapers, magazines, fiction, non-fiction ? ....

(3) Do you enjoy reading ? ....

(4) Can you read fast and easily ? ....

(5) Can you read non-stop for an hour or more ?
....

(6) Do you remember what you read ? ....

(7) Do you lose yourself while reading or are you easily disturbed by noises, conversations or visual distractions ?
....

(8) If you encounter an unfamiliar word while reading, do you reach for the dictionary or carry on ? ....

(9) If you do not understand a phrase or a sentence, do you read again and again ? ....

(10) Do you overlook words or letters and therefore do you have to read the sentence again ? ....

(11) Following reading or writing, do you suffer from eye-strain or headache ? If yes, after how much time ? ....

> **Note :**
> **Persons with fixated-central visual style –**
> * enjoy reading and if given a choice, prefer it to an outdoor walk,
> * can read for hours at a time, anywhere, any time with minimal distraction,
> * read smoothly, with good speed, concentration and retention,
> * display good visual memory of the passages read,
> * can sit, almost motionless, for hours while reading.
>
> **Persons with peripheral-scanning visual style –**
> * dislike reading and prefer long-range or far-point visual tasks,
> * tend to read only when required but not for pleasure,
> * become restless following prolonged reading, experience concentration lapses or nervous tension,
> * often skim articles, read paragraphs out of order, are generally impatient and turn to the end of the section to know "what happens",
> * have not-so-good visual memory and cannot easily retain the information that has been read.

(B) Television viewing :

(1) For how many hours a day do you view television ? ....

(2) Do you look at the T.V. intensely or perform other tasks or converse simultaneously ? ....

(3) Do you sit close to the T.V. or reasonably far ? ....

(4) While watching the T.V., do you rely as much on your ears as on your eyes ? ....

(5) While viewing the T.V., do you prefer complete darkness in the room or do you keep a light on ? ....

> **Note :** Generally, persons with a fixated-central visual style sit quite close to the T.V., prefer a small screen and a dark room and watch with great concentration.
>
> Persons with a scanning-peripheral visual style sit far away from the T.V., prefer a larger screen and a lighted room, may simultaneously perform other tasks and possess a not-so-good memory of things seen.

(C) Hobbies :

(1) Which hobbies have you cultivated ? ....

(2) How do you pass your free time ? Collect stamps or coins ? read ? listen to music ? play outdoor sports ? go for outings ? ....

> **Note** : Persons with fixated-central visual style are usually seen to possess hobbies requiring close-range vision. They prefer collecting stamps or coins to gardening or swimming.
>
> Persons with scanning-peripheral visual style usually cultivate outdoor hobbies. They prefer playing badminton or hockey to playing table tennis or cards.

(D) Driving :

(1) Are you relaxed when you drive ? Or become tense ? ....

(2) Do you enjoy driving ? ....

(3) Do you pay attention to developing traffic patterns way ahead of you ? ....

(4) Do you have trouble shifting your focus from far to near or near to far ? ....

(5) Do you pay attention to what is going on to your right and left ? ....

(6) Do you look into the rear-view mirror frequently ? ....

(7) Do oncoming cars make you tense ? ....

(8) Do you find night driving difficult or tiring ? ....

> **Note :**
> **Persons with fixated-central visual style —**
> * find that night driving is tiring,
> * tend to sit forward and view straight ahead,
> * have trouble with driving at dusk or night,
> * are rendered tense or taken by surprise by oncoming traffic,
> * do not automatically take into account the traffic on the left or the right.

Persons with scanning-peripheral visual style –
* enjoy driving and are therefore relaxed,
* are less troubled by night-driving,
* have endurance for long drives,
* enjoy sizing up developing traffic patterns far ahead of them,
* sit back and view the panorama.

(3) Personality :

(A) Nature :

(1) Are you shy ? ....

(2) Do you suffer from an inferiority complex ? ....

(3) Are you at ease while talking to elders or well-known persons ? ....

(4) Do you usually consider yourself less intelligent or successful than others ? ....

(5) Do you hesitate to use or display your talents ? ....

(6) Could you speak or sing if pushed onto a stage ? ....

(7) Do you become unduly self-conscious in a crowd ? ....

(8) Are you an introvert ? ....

(9) Can you get familiar with strangers soon ? ....

(10) Can you make friends easily ? ....

How many fast friends do you have ? ....

(11) Do you like solitude ? ....

(12) If given a choice, will you prefer reading in solitude to chit-chatting with friends ? ....

(13) Are you unduly polite and well-mannered ? ....

Note :
Persons with fixated-central visual style are usually shy, introverts, reserved and unduly self-conscious. They usually suffer from an inferiority complex, lack confidence, feel nervous in a crowd or while talking to superior persons, love solitude and have only a few friends.

Persons with scanning-peripheral visual style are usually bold, confident, extroverts and happy-go-lucky. They do not hesitate to talk to strangers, make friends easily, feel quite at ease while talking to superior persons and dislike solitude.

(B) Approach to life :

(1) How well can you face a difficult situation ? ....

(2) Can you take an immediate decision and act accordingly ? ....

(3) Do you lose too much time in thinking ? ....

(4) Do you try to run away from difficulties ? ....

(5) Do you usually make compromises or settle for less ? ....

Note :

Persons with fixated-central visual style usually find difficulty in reaching a decision in the face of a difficult situation, or they cannot put the decision into practice. They make compromises quite readily.

Persons with scanning-peripheral visual style not only take quick decisions but even put them into practice. They do not lose undue time in thinking and do not compromise easily.

(C) Occupation and approach to work :

(1) What is your occupation ? ....

(2) Does your occupation entail a lot of near-point visual work ? ....

(3) What type of work would you prefer, if given a choice ? ....

(4) Do you work methodically and zealously ? ....

(5) Do you always complete the task you undertake ?
....

Note :

Persons with fixated-central visual style prefer sedentary occupations entailing long periods of near-point work. They sit for hours without moving. They are very methodical in their work and usually complete the work they undertake.

Persons with scanning-peripheral visual style are usually businessmen and seldom professionals like doctors or chartered accountants. In other words, they are found in occupations which call for team-work. They prefer a more active life and dislike sedentary jobs. They are somewhat careless in work, less methodical and lacking in concentration. They do not necessarily complete the task they undertake.

(D) Education :

(1) How many years have you spent in studying ?

....

(2) What are your educational qualifications ? ....

(3) Did you earn good marks in school/college ? ....

(4) Were you a favourite with teachers ? ....

Note :

Persons with fixated-central visual style spend many years in studying and are educationally well-qualified. In school/college, they work very hard to secure a good percentage of marks in the examinations.

Persons with scanning-peripheral visual style are less interested in reading or writing. Hence they do not secure high marks in school/college examinations.

(E) Sports :

(1) Do you actively and regularly participate in sports ?

....

(2) Are you more interested in playing than in studying ?

....

(3) Which sports do you like : indoor or outdoor ?

....

(4) From among outdoor sports, do you like such sports as provide individual opportunities (viz. tennis, cricket) or which call for team-work (viz. football, hockey) ? ....

(5) Would you prefer playing a game to reading an interesting book ? ....

(6) Do you play such games as require fast running ? Are your reflexes fast enough ? ....

> **Note :**
> Persons with a fixated-central visual style usually display a lack of interest in outdoor sports. If at all, they play such games as provide chances for individual success or which do not entail much physical labour. They would prefer reading a book to playing a fast game.
> Persons with a scanning-peripheral visual style are sportsmen and athletes. They have a great liking for fast, outdoor games. Among outdoor games, they play such games as require a team effort. They prefer playing in the open to reading a book at home.

(F) Social Life :

(1) Do you participate in social functions ? ....

(2) Do you like social gatherings and crowds ? ....

> **Note :**
> Persons with a fixated-central visual style generally like solitude, keep away from social functions and fell awkward of nervous in a gathering or a crowd.
> Persons with scanning-peripheral visual style enjoy social functions and gatherings and always look forward to meeting friends and relatives.

CONCLUSION

For efficient and trouble-free sight, a well-balanced visual style is necessary. An undue inclination towards a particular style produces or aggravates a host of problems. For example, the fixated-central style may, over the years, give rise to or worsen myopia and exophoria; the scanning-peripheral visual style is, many a time, found associated with hypermetropia and esophoria.

If your answers to the questions and tests described in this chapter indicate that you possess a particular visual style, you should strive to avoid misuse of your eyes and bring about a gradual modification in your style. For example, if your's is a fixated-central visual style, you will make it a point to look out of the window every now and then while reading or writing; besides, you will take a break after every half an hour of near-point work. If you become aware of the fact that you miss or overlook details when walking down the street, you can consciously focus your attention and your eyes on objects that lie on your sides, which you usually ignored earlier. Remember that the transition may prove to be a bit difficult. But with perseverance, you will be able to modify your visual style sooner or later and increase your visual potential.

In fact, moulding your child's visual style correctly is a better way of attaining the goal of strong eyes and flexible vision, for the whole life.

What to do for a child ?

Spend a few days watching your child; notice its reading habits, general approach to tasks, levels of concentration etc. Then fill out the same questionnaire given earlier in this chapter.

Remember that children upto the age of six or seven are naturally scanning-peripheral. This style begins to get modified, as the child learns to read and write. Hypermetropia may delay and myopia may hasten this transition towards a more balanced style.

Once you have determined your child's visual style, take time to explain to it in simple words, the concept of vision-training. In general terms, let your child know that you are going to work with it to help it get the most out of all the visual activities it undertakes : sports, games, school-work, reading etc. Do not criticize the child for its way of approaching visual tasks. Offer gentle suggestions.

In our practice, we see a lot of kids who need vision training. To get their full participation and co-operation, it is necessary to explain to them what it is all about and why they are going to do it. They must learn to recognise their visual style so that they can correct their bad habits. For example, if we were talking to a child with a fixated-central style, we would say : *"It seems that you look very hard at things, too intensely, with too much concentration. That is why your eyes tire. You do not notice all that is going on around you."*

To a child who is excessively scanning-peripheral, we would say : *"You really notice a lot of what is going on around you. But you have trouble paying keen attention to one thing at a time. There are times when you move your eyes around when they should be held steady, e.g., while reading. This may make it hard for you to learn."*

---

7. SELF-ASSESSMENT : PART TWO

After determining the nature to our visual style and personality, we should find out if we have specific visual defects.

This chapter contains a series of self-assessment procedures which would make us aware of our present visual status and existing visual errors like nearsightedness, farsightedness, astigmatism, amblyopia, muscle imbalances, fusion problems or suppression.

These tests are not designed to take the place of professional eye-care. They provide us with a clue to visual defect present in our eyes and form a part of an overall vision-hygiene programme.

Self-assessment tests reveal potential vision problems so that we can seek good professional advice and care.

Self-assessment tests work in conjunction with a doctor's diagnosis. The most effective way of handling vision problems is to combine professional therapy with a deep personal commitment to self-care.

After each test, there is an evaluation note. At the end of the chapter, we collate this information with the information about visual style which we gathered in the previous chapter. Our conclusions guide us in selecting the vision-training programme that will solve our specific problems effectively.

(1) Myopia (Nearsightedness) : Myopia is a visual defect in which a person cannot see distant objects clearly. The near vision is usually quite good, as the name suggests.

In myopia, parallel rays of light coming from distant objects are bent more than normally inside the eye, so that they come to a focus some distance ahead of the retina (the screen of the eye). Hence the image formed on the retina is fuzzy and the person sees blurred images.

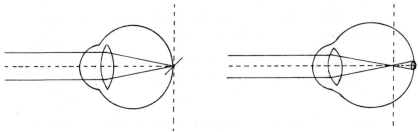

Fig. 7.1

Nearsightedness is on the rise throughout the world. We are fast becoming a generation of handicapped persons. The age at which this defect begins is going down from adolescence to the pre-school years and the number it affects keeps going up, especially among the educated.

Traditional medicine clings to the idea that myopia is the result of a hereditory predisposition for an elongation of the eyeball, and furthermore that there is nothing we can do except resort to stronger and stronger glasses as the defect advances.

If myopia is inherited, from whom did we inherit it ? Why weren't our forefathers nearsighted to the same degree as we are ? Nearsightedness is practically unknown where book-learning is not prized. In our culture, the city-bred folk are more prone to myopia than their country cousins; honours students and graduates have higher incidence of myopia than school dropouts.

If myopia were simply a condition which happened to some and not to others, the following statistical variables would not follow this orderly and predictable pattern :

* Before the age of ten years, approximately three to four per cent of the population are nearsighted. By the time children complete middle-school education, ten to fifteen per cent are nearsighted. At the end of high school education, the number has jumped to twenty per cent. And at the end of college education, the incidence has soared to thirty to thirty-five per cent. None of our other senses is prone to such an overwhelming and rapid deterioration.

* At the U. S. Naval Academy, the new entrants have good visual-acuity since it is a basic requirement for admission. By graduation, a high percentage becomes myopic.

* Among children of migrant workers, who are never at school for any great length of time, the incidence of myopia remains a fairly constant six per cent. Farm children who spend more time outdoors, gazing restfully at the horizon, have a lesser incidence of myopia than city kids.

* In a survey of Eskimo families, only 2 out of 130 persons who could not read or write showed myopia; yet among their children who were attending school and eating a Western diet, approximately 65 per cent were nearsighted. This happened in a single generation in a population known to be somewhat farsighted. When the grandparents were examined, they showed the same absence of myopia as their progeny, i.e., the parents of the nearsighted group. If it were true that vision is inherited, the grandchildren should have been farsighted. But, on the contrary, they were nearsighted. Although this example shows a massive reversal in a single generation, the erroneous assumption that nearsightedness is hereditory still persists.

* In Japan, before World War II, the figures for myopia were quite high. During the difficult years of the war, academic education was neglected; when the fighting stopped and the schools were about to re-open, it was discovered that myopia among the student population had nearly halved. As years went by and education continued, the incidence of myopia rose again. It has now shot back to the pre-war figures.

We could go on and on quoting studies and statistics, but they all tell the same story : as literacy rises, so does myopia. Yet books continue to be written stating that myopia is inherited – the result of a lengthening of the eyeball. But why did the eyeball stretch out ? The study on Eskimos mentioned above alone would seem to disprove the heredity factor. It appears that we are doing something to ourselves to cause the rapid increase in the incidence of myopia.

The propounders of the genetic theory argue that children of nearsighted parents are mostly nearsighted. But this probably is the result of certain personality traits : ambition, inhibition and scholarliness. Dr. Francis Young, a psychologist at Washington State University, makes an interesting analogy to illustrate the lack of logic in incriminating heredity for myopia : if an English-speaking person marries an English-speaking person, they will give birth to a child who also becomes an English-speaking person. But is the English inherited ?

Myopia does not occur overnight; it comes on slowly and may go unnoticed until a student complains that he can't see what is written on the blackboard or that his eyes tire easily. As we have explained, it appears to be caused by overworking specific eye-muscles to focus at near-point. The human eye is at rest while looking into the distance.

The eye under constant stress tries to send a warning sign : pain. *"Hey you, I am tired. Why don't you stop reading for a while ?........"* Athletes talk about their pain; the diligent student simply presses on to the next page.

Eventually, the eye grows accustomed to the strain, gives up sending pain messages, but grumbles when asked to see a far : *"Why do we need to bother with that ? I can do this close-range work for you so well........"*

After a long period of reading, there will be a slight amount of temporary blurring when shifting the focus to a distant point. *"What is this ? You want to look at the sunset now ? Why are you making my life so hard ?....,"* the eyes will say.

If the stress caused by close-range work continues at the same rate and the student marches right along–reading,

reading and reading–the focussing ability of distant objects weakens to the point where there is an actual loss of visual acuity that can be measured on a chart. *"I tried to tell you I need rest; but what did I get from you ? Another book. Okay, I am getting used to the idea."*

And as the near-point work continues, and the student works hard to stay ahead of his colleagues, the eye-muscles eventually lock into place; the pressure has been too great to overcome. The eyeball lengthens and the image the eye receives comes to a focus in front of the retina, rather than on it, as in a normal eye. *"Okay, you win. Now I have become perfectly suited to your type of life–the life of a scholar. Of course, something had to be sacrificed, and that is my ability to see clearly at distance."*

Sounds like a series of cliches ? Well, the psychologists, psychiatrists and other researchers who have studied the problem of myopia say these cliches are more or less true. They are generalisations of course, but still statistically on the graph.

It has been stated earlier that myopia is related to specific personality traits. Again and again, myopes have been found to be introverts, introspective, shy, meticulous, disinclined to participation in sports and having a marked preference for sedentary activities. They are self-centred, dogmatic, diligent and in control of their emotions. In choosing an occupation, the myope tends to select those in which individual achievement, rather than team effort, is necessary. Lonely intellectual pursuits such as those of authors, journalists, doctors, architects and scholars are favoured.

Testing for nearsightedness :

Props : Distant-vision testing chart provided at the end of this book.

Glasses : Do not use glasses.

Routine :

(1) Place or hang the chart on the wall at eye level. Make sure that the chart is well illuminated.

(2) Measure five feet from the chart; mark it. Measure ten feet from the chart; mark it. Measure twenty feet from the chart; mark it.

(3) Stand at the twenty-feet mark.

(4) Cover the left eye with the left palm.

(5) Read the chart from top to bottom, slowly. Do not make undue efforts or squeeze the eyes while reading. Make a note of the number of lines or letters you can read correctly.

(6) Step forward to the ten-feet mark. Repeat the procedure. Make a note of how many lines or letters you can read correctly.

(7) Then step forward to the five-feet mark. Repeat the procedure. Make a note of the number of lines or letters you can read correctly.

(8) If you cannot clearly see lines or letters even from five feet, advance towards the chart until you can. Make a note of the distance from the chart.

(9) Finally, repeat the entire routine with the left eye, keeping the right eye covered with the right palm.

Observation :

Right eye :

(1) From twenty feet, I could read .... lines correctly.

(2) From ten feet, I could read .... lines correctly.

(3) From five feet, I could read .... lines correctly.

(4) I could read all letters clearly from a distance of .... feet.

Left eye⁻:

(1) From twenty feet, I could read .... lines correctly.

(2) From ten feet, I could read .... lines correctly.

(3) From five feet, I could read .... lines correctly.

(4) I could read all letters clearly from a distance of .... feet.

Evaluation : Clear vision at twenty feet means that you have no or negligible myopia. Clear vision at ten feet indicates mild (low) myopia. Clear vision at five feet indicates moderate myopia. Clear vision at less than five feet indicates high myopia.

> **Note :** The visual acuity of the two eyes may turn out to be different, i.e., the visual status or refracting power of the two eyes is not necessarily similar. If one eye has no myopia and the other eye is myopic or if one eye has a lesser degree and the other eye a greater degree of myopia (or any particular visual defect), the condition is known as **anisometropia**. Anisometropia is often associated with other visual or ocular defects like fusion problems, suppression of the vision of the weaker eye and latent squint (heterophoria). Tests to uncover these defects have been described later in this chapter.

(2) Hypermetropia (Farsightedness) : Hypermetropia is a visual defect in which the distant vision is usually quite good (as the name suggests) but the person experiences difficulty while performing a near-point task. However, if the defect is severe, even the distant vision may be subnormal. Even in such cases, the difficulty for work at near distance is much greater than that for work at a distance.

Hypermetropia which develops at or around the age of forty years is given a special name : **'Presbyopia'.** Presbyopia develops because of a gradual hardening of the crystalline lens of the eye, with advancing age.

In hypermetropia, parallel rays of light coming from distant objects, on entering the eye, are bent less than normal, so that they come to a focus some distance behind the retina. Divergent rays of light coming from nearby objects come to a focus farther behind the retina.

Our eye has a certain power to increase the bending (convergence) of light rays entering the eye. This power is called the 'accommodative power'. It is because of accommodation that a hypermetrope usually sees distant objects quite clearly. However, the accommodative power may be insufficient to enable the person to see near objects clearly.

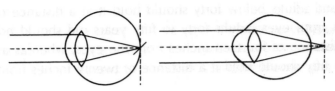

Fig. 7.2

The constant use of accommodation taxes the muscles inside the eye and many a time gives rise to symptoms like eye-fatigue, eye-strain and headaches.

While the evidence clearly indicates that myopia is the result of environmental factors, the causes of hypermetropia are not so clear.

The behaviour associated with farsightedness is almost opposite to that associated with myopia. Research has shown that farsighted individuals tend to be more concerned about tomorrow than the here and the now. They are usually extroverts, confident, less meticulous or diligent and tend to show off their emotions. They like overall organisation and structure but tend to gloss over details. They choose professions where teamwork is essential, e.g., business. They are often the centre of activity—but on the playing field rather than the chess club or the table-tennis court. They enjoy team sports like hockey or football.

Testing for farsightedness :

Props : Both near as well as distant eye-sight testing charts provided at the end of this book.

Glasses : Do not use glasses.

Routine :

(1) Place or hang the distant-sight testing chart on the wall at eye level.

(2) Measure twenty feet from the chart and mark it.

(3) Stand or sit at the twenty-feet mark.

(4) Hold the near-sight testing chart in your hands. Children and adults below forty should hold it at a distance of six inches from eyes, adults forty to fifty years old should hold it at a distance of fourteen inches from the eyes, whereas adults above fifty should hold it a distance of twenty inches from the eyes.

(5) Cover the left eye with the left palm.

(6) Look at the near-sight testing chart. Focus if possible. Can the smallest print be easily read ?

(7) Shift the gaze to the distant-sight testing chart. Are all the letters quite clear ? Keep looking at the distant chart for a while.

(8) Shift the gaze quickly back to the near chart.

(9) Note the focal shift. Is the smallest print clear ? Does the print become clear after some time ? Do you have to move the near chart slightly away to be able to read the smallest print ?

(10) Would you say that reading the distant chart is easier for you than reading the near chart ?

(11) Repeat the entire procedure with the left eye, keeping the right eye covered with the right palm.

Observation :

Right eye :

(1) I could read all / only some lines of the distant chart clearly.

(2) The letters of the distant chart were clear immediately/after some time.

(3) I could / could not read the smallest print of the near chart clearly.

(4) After shifting the gaze from the distant to the near chart, the print was immediately (a) clear or (b) clear after some time or (c) clear only on moving the near chart away.

(5) I could read at distance/near more easily than near/ distance.

Left eye :

(1) I could read all/only some lines of the distant chart clearly.

(2) The letters of the distant chart were clear immediately/after some time.

(3) I could/could not read the smallest print on the near chart clearly.

(4) After shifting the gaze from the distant to the near chart, the print was immediately (a) clear or (b) clear after some time or (c) clear only on moving the near chart away.

(5) I could read at distance / near more easily than near / distance.

Evaluation : If you can immediately see clearly distant as well as near charts, you probably do not suffer from hypermetropia. After shifting the gaze from distant to near chart, if the smallest print becomes clear only after some time or on moving the chart away, or if the smallest print is not clear, you have low to moderate hypermetropia. If you can't read even the distant chart clearly and if you have greater difficulty for near than for distance, you have high hypermetropia. If your age is about 40 years and if you have recently started experiencing difficulty for near, you have a special type of hypermetropia, termed presbyopia.

> **Note :** The visual status of the two eyes is not necessarily similar. One eye may be normal and the other farsighted, or, one eye may have a lesser degree of farsightedness and the other may have a greater degree of farsightedness. Such a condition is called anisometropia. Anisometropia is often associated with other visual or ocular defects like fusion problems, suppression of the vision of the weaker eye and latent squint. Tests to detect the presence or absence of these defects have been described later in this chapter.

(3) Astigmatism : Astigmatism is a visual defect which is caused by an irregularity in the surface of either the cornea or the crystalline lens. When corneal or lenticular surface is regular, all the light rays entering the eye form a point focus. But if corneal or lenticular surface is irregular (i.e., steeper in one plane and flatter in the other), the light rays entering the eyes form two separate focal lines. This has been diagrammatically presented below. A person with astigmatism usually sees a part (meridian) of an object more clearly than another part (meridian) situated at a right angle to the former part.

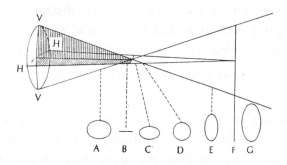

Fig. 7.3

VV—the vertical meridian of cornea which is more curved (steeper) than HH—the horizontal meridian of cornea. Note that the rays of light striking the cornea along its vertical meridian are bent more acutely than those striking the cornea along its horizontal meridian. Hence instead of a point-focus, two focal lines are formed (at B and F).

Understanding how astigmatism develops can be instrumental in preventing or treating it. If posture is tilted or the face mis-shapen, the eyes will attempt to compensate for the distortion and try their best to maintain a correct balance, straining some muscles and relaxing others.

How a physical imbalance can lead to optical distortions can be easily understood if we imagine that the body is composed of triangles balancing on top of one another. If one of the triangles is not balanced, the others won't be either.

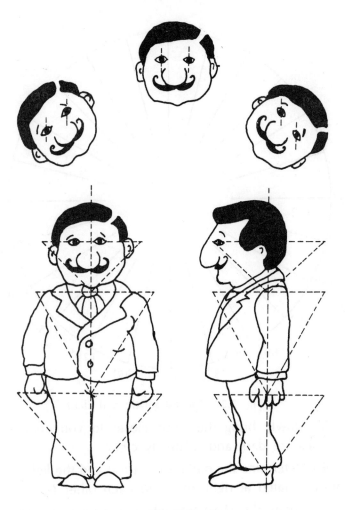

Fig. 7.4

Besides blurred vision and eye-strain, astigmatism often results in headaches.

Testing for astigmatism :

Props : Dial chart given on page 54.

Glasses : Do not use glasses.

Routine :

(1) Cover the left eye with the left palm.

(2) Hold the dial chart in the right hand and stretch the arm so that the chart comes to lie far away from the eye.

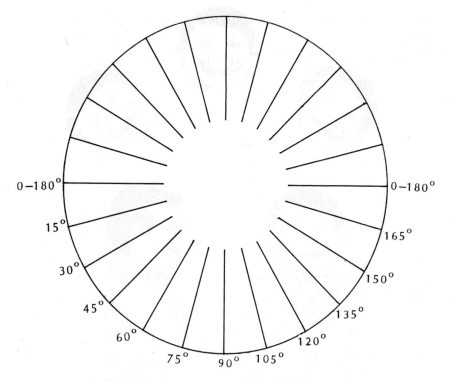

Fig. 7.5 : The astigmatic dial chart

(3) Slowly bring the chart closer to you until at least some lines are dark and relatively clear.

(4) Determine the darkest (clearest) and the lightest lines. Are they situated at right angles to each other ?

(5) Rotate the chart through ninety degrees. The spatial location of the most clear and most blurred lines should remain the same.

(6) Repeat the entire routine with the left eye, keeping the right eye covered with the right palm.

Evaluation : If all the lines appear equally clear, it indicates an absence of astigmatism. If the line of a particular meridian appears darker than the rest and if the line perpendicular to it appears the least clear, it is an indication of astigmatism. The greater the difference in tone between the clear and the blurred lines, the greater the degree of astigmatism.

(4) **Suppression** : We have two eyes, the retina of each eye forming an image of its own. Yet, when we look at an object, we do not see it double because our brain processes the two images and fuses them into one. Such fusion is possible only if the two images are almost similar in size and clarity. Our brain cannot fuse two considerably dissimilar images. The images on the two retinae will be dissimilar if the refractive power (visual status) of the two eyes is vastly different (i.e., if one eye is normal or has a slight defect and the other has a greater defect requiring a glass) or if one of the eyes is a crossed eye (i.e., it has turned in or out, so that noncorresponding areas of two retinae are stimulated). Dissimilar images are sources of confusion for the brain. The brain, therefore, concentrates only on one (better) image and ignores the other. This phenomenon is called suppression.

The suppressed eye can perform by itself when necessary, so that this condition is not discovered when the victim covers the other eye. The person is not usually aware that he is not seeing with both eyes together.

The vision of a person with suppression in one eye could be thought of as one dimensional. He finds it difficult to judge the location of an object in space correctly. He bumps into things or knocks over glasses. He does not know or understand what is wrong or missing and why he is so clumsy. H. G. Wells has written in his autobiography that he believed his unbalanced or uneven vision, good in one eye but poor in the other, had prevented him from becoming a better writer.

If suppression is not corrected or treated in time, the suppressed eye gradually loses its power of seeing and becomes amblyopic. An amblyopic eye is a lazy eye which cannot be fully awakened (i.e., its vision cannot be corrected) even with appropriate glasses. Amblyopia has been described in greater details later in this chapter.

Testing for suppression :

Props : A thin rope (string) twelve feet long, three buttons or beads that will thread securely, but not too tightly, on the rope.

Glasses : Perform the routine first without and then with glasses on.

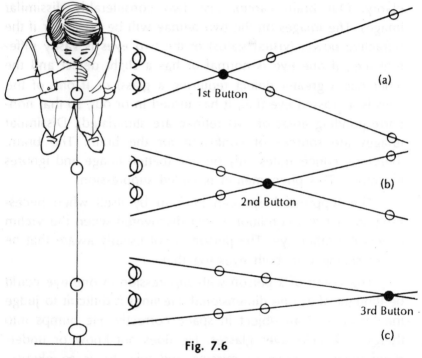

Fig. 7.6

Routine :

(1) Tie one end of the string to a door-knob. Place buttons on the string at distances of six inches, eighteen inches and four feet from the door-knob.

(2) Stand twelve feet from the door-knob. Hold the string taut against the tip of your nose.

(3) With both the eyes, look at the hole of the button closest to you.

(4) You should see two strings, crossing exactly in the button-hole [see figure (a) above].

(5) Work to direct both your eyes exactly at the centre of the button-hole.

(6) Are both the strings visible ?

Is one string less distinct than the other ? ....

Which one ? ....

Is one of the strings only partially visible ? ....

Which one ? ....

Does one string disappear completely ? ....

Which one ? ....

(7) Repeat the routine with each of the remaining buttons on the string.

Evaluation : If whole lengths of the two strings are clearly visible and they cross at the button-hole you are looking at, both your eyes are seeing simultaneously and the vision of neither of the eyes is being suppressed by the brain.

If one of the two strings is less distinct than the other (even when you are wearing correct glasses) or if one of the strings disappears partially or completely, the vision of one of your eyes is being suppressed by the brain. Suppression of the right eye is indicated by indistinctness or disappearance of the left string and vice versa. Just indistinctness indicates mild suppression, partial disappearance indicates marked suppression and total disappearance indicates total suppression of the vision of a particular eye.

(5) **Amblyopia (Lazy eye) :** Amblyopia is a visual defect characterised by subnormal vision which cannot be corrected with glasses, in spite of an absence of demonstrable disease. Amblyopia or laziness is the natural consequence of long-term disuse or suppression of an eye. It should be noted that severe congenital visual defects in both eyes, if not corrected in time, may result in laziness of both the eyes.

The physical effects of amblyopia are similar to those of suppression of an eye.

Testing for amblyopia :

Props : Distant eye-sight testing chart.

Glasses : If glasses are required for distant vision, wear them.

Routine :

(1) Sit or stand twenty feet from the chart.

(2) Cover the left eye with the left palm.

(3) Looking at the distant chart, can you read at least six lines clearly ?

(4) If six lines are not visible, see through a minute hole (pinhole), made in a small piece of cardboard. Are six lines clearly visible now ?

(5) Repeat the entire routine with the left eye, keeping the right eye covered with the right palm.

Evaluation : Inability to read at least six lines clearly through the pinhole points to a possibility of amblyopia.

Vision not clear previously, but becoming clear on peeping through the pin-hole indicates a change in spectacle power and not amblyopia.

It should be noted that subnormal vision, not improving on seeing through a pinhole, may also be a result of some eye-disease.

(6) **Convergence Insufficiency :** When looking at distance, our eyes are almost parallel, i.e., both point straight ahead. However, when looking at a near object, they come close to each other to maintain binocular fixation. Such simultaneous turning of the two eyes towards the nose is called convergence. Efficient convergence is necessary for trouble-free near-point work. Convergence insufficiency gives rise to eye-strain, headaches, watering and intermittent double vision (jumbling together of letters) following a certain period of near-point work like reading or writing.

Testing for convergence efficiency :

Props : A small rectangular card with a dark yet fine vertical line along its breadth (see picture below).

Glasses : Do not use glasses.

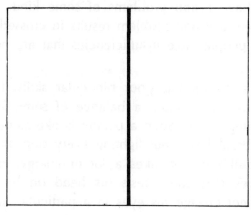

Fig. 7.7

Routine :

(1) Hold the card in your hand, with the arm extended.

(2) Keep looking at the vertical line with both the eyes.

(3) Slowly bring the card towards your eyes; stop when the card is six inches from your eyes.

(4) Does the line appear single or double ?

Evaluation : A person with good convergence power sees a single line even when the card is held as close as six inches from the eyes.

If the line appears double as the card approaches the inner limit of six inches, your convergence is insufficient. This means that both your eyes are not pointing towards the line.

The greater the insufficiency of convergence, the greater will be the distance of the card from the eyes when the line starts appearing double.

(7) **Fusion Problems :** We have two eyes, each of which forms its own image. Yet we do not see an object double because our brain fuses the two images into one. Thus, we possess 'binocular single vision'. It is because of good fusion that our vision is three dimensional and we are able to locate an object in space accurately.

It is an alarming fact that a full seventy per cent of the population have fusion problems of some kind. At its most severe degree, a fusion problem results in crossed eye; but a great many people have insufficiencies that are not so apparent.

When a person has poor binocular skills, he is under constant stress to maintain a balance of some sort to keep from becoming worse. Such a person is like someone on the verge of a breakdown, but fighting every step of the way to maintain equilibrium. It takes a lot of energy. He probably rubs his eyes frequently, rests his head on his arm when writing, cannot engage his eyes in a particular activity for a very long time and experiences sporadic double vision.

Without good depth perception resulting out of inefficient binocular vision, a person has difficulty in catching a ball, feels quite uneasy walking over a bridge or standing at the edge of a terrace and needs to hold onto a railing when going down steps because he is uncertain about the space in front of him and has difficulty in judging precisely where the edge of the step is.

Testing for fusion problems :

Props : A small torch or pen-light (candle flame can be used instead), a 3 x 5 inch card, a dark room.

Glasses : Perform the routine first without and then with glasses.

Routine :

(1) Sit about 15 feet away from the light or the candle.

(2) Look at the light or the candle-flame with both the eyes.

(3) Hold the card in front of any one eye so as to occlude its vision (the eye, however, should be kept open).

(4) Look at the light with the uncovered eye for ten counts.

(5) Keeping the gaze fixed on the light, rapidly remove the card to expose the covered eye.

(6) Do you momentarily see two lights ? Do the two lights merge immediately or after some time ?

Evaluation : Double vision (seeing two lights) is an indication of a certain degree of fusion problem.

If the two lights merge immediately, the fusion problem is slight.

If the two lights merge after some time, you have moderate fusion problem.

If the two lights merge after two seconds or more or if an effort is required on your part to bring about their fusion, you have marked fusion problem.

> **Notes :** (1) Whichever eye is covered, the result turns out to be the same; that is to say that the problem is not specific to a particular eye.
>
> (2) The problem gets aggravated and therefore can be elicited more easily when the eyes are tired (say following a session of reading or writing) or when a person is sick.

(8) **Heterophoria (Latent or Hidden squint) :** Seeing with both the eyes together yields definite advantages—a person's vision is more clear and three dimensional and his field of vision is enlarged.

For binocular single vision, both the eyes should be accurately directed towards the object of attention. For this, the various eye-muscles have to work in a co-ordinated and balanced manner.

Many a time, a particular set of eye muscles is weak as compared to the others and, therefore, the eyes have a tendency to deviate in a particular direction. However, to gain the advantages of binocular vision, the brain keeps such tendency for squinting under check, by constantly overworking the weak muscles.

Such a condition in which the tendency to squinting is not allowed to become manifest and the two eyes are usually maintained parallel and straight by a constant effort from the brain is called heterophoria or hidden squint.

Such constant overworking of the weak muscles has its deleterious effects. A person with a hidden squint commonly suffers from eye-strain, undue eye-fatigue, headaches and occasional double vision.

When the muscles that move eyes inward (nasally) are weak (and therefore the eyes tend to deviate outward), the condition is called exophoria. If the muscles moving the eyes outward are weak, the condition is called esophoria. The incidence of upward or downward deviation (hidden vertical squint) is very low.

Testing for heterophoria :

Props : Distant vision testing chart, a 3 x 5 inch card.

Glasses : Use glasses if needed to see clearly.

Routine :

(1) Sit or stand fifteen feet from the distant chart.

(2) Select a small letter of the chart and look steadily at it with both the eyes.

(3) Cover the right eye with the small card so as to occlude its vision; however, the eye should be kept open behind the card.

(4) Move the card very quickly from your right eye to your left eye without moving your head and ensuring that during the process, the right eye vision is not obstructed.

(5) Does the letter appear to 'jump' or move when you change your gaze from your left eye to the right eye ? In which direction did the letter move–from left to right (i.e., from nose toward the right ear) or vice versa ? What was the extent of the movement ?

Evaluation : If the target letter does not move, you do not have a hidden squint, i.e., the muscle-balance is good.

If the letter moves or jumps from the left to the right direction, you have exophoria and if it jumps from the right to the left, you have esophoria.

If the letter moves less than one inch in either direction, your phoria is extremely slight, indeed insignificant.

If the letter moves one to three inches, you have a slight phoria; if the letter moves three to six inches, you have a moderate phoria and if the letter moves more than six inches, you have severe phoria.

SELF-ASSESSMENT RESULTS AT A GLANCE

Yes / No

1. I think I am developing nearsightedness.

2. I am nearsighted.

3. One of my eyes is more myopic than the other.

4. I am farsighted.

5. One of my eyes is more farsighted than the other.

6. I have presbyopia.

7. I have astigmatism in the right eye.

8. I have astigmatism in the left eye.

9. The vision of my right eye is mildly/markedly/ totally suppressed.

10. The vision of my left eye is mildly/markedly/ totally suppressed.

11. My eyes converge insufficiently.

12. I have slight / moderate/marked fusion problems.

13. I have slight / moderate/severe exophoria.

14. I have slight / moderate/severe esophoria.

Thus, I require to perform exercises for my following problems :

1. ....

2. ....

3. ....

....

....

8. VISION TRAINING EXERCISES

This chapter describes various exercises that either train the vision, strengthen the eyes or help in some other way like increasing the focal flexibility or overcoming muscle-imbalances, suppression or laziness. Some exercises are meant specially for specific visual or occular defects; others are general exercises that can be performed by any person, whether he or she has weak eyes or good eyes.

There are some basic guidelines to be kept in mind while performing any exercise :

(1) First carefully read and understand the method of performing the exercise. Understand the steps and the goal involved; keep the necessary charts and props handy.

(2) Generally, use glasses only when absolutely necessary to do the exercise. You want to extend your visual limits and make your eyes work on their own. Use glasses during an exercise only if specific instructions to do so have been given.

(3) Make sure that you do the exercises in non-glaring, full light. Have targets and charts brightly illuminated at all times.

(4) Whenever instructed to close one or both of the eyes, do so gently. Gently place the palm of the same side on the eye, when its vision is to be occluded.

(5) While doing an exercise, do not strain your eyes. You are striving for relaxed, responsive focal power. Do not struggle to accomplish the exercise because that is counterproductive. You will have a greater success in seeing clearly if you do not work too hard or strain your eyes to achieve goals. The eyes respond to restrained guidance, not intense force.

(6) Even if you have trouble with an exercise, stick with it. Do not abandon an exercise even if the schedule indicates you should discontinue it or replace it with some other exercise.

(7) As you go through the four week training programme, your eye-sight or eye-efficiency will slowly improve. Use the evaluation sections that follow each exercise to keep track of your progress.

(8) As you become more and more proficient with a particular exercise, adjust the distance of near and/or far objects (targets) to encounter stiffer challenges progressively.

(9) Do not forget to rest your eyes after every exercise and finally at the end of the whole exercise programme. There are a number of ways to rest the eyes; they have been described in chapter 5.

(10) It is desirable to paste the various charts on cardboards. They are then easier to handle and last longer.

(11) Generally speaking, early morning is the best time to perform exercises. The whole-day work may tire the eyes and exercising the tired eyes is undesirable.

(12) If you do not have enough time to do all the exercises together, you may do some (difficult ones) in the morning and the rest in the evening.

GENERAL EXERCISES TO MAKE EYES AND VISION STRONG AND EFFICIENT

Number one : Sinhasana (Sinha Mudra or Lion Pose)

Aim : To preserve or improve eyesight.

Props : None.

Method : First assume the 'Vajrasana' posture (see diagrams below).

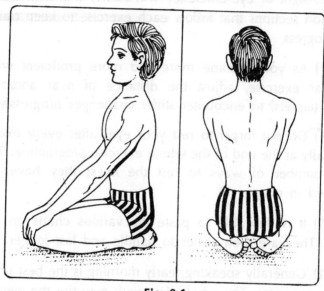

Fig. 8.1

Now open the mouth wide, bring the tongue out as much as possible and look upward (see the photograph below).

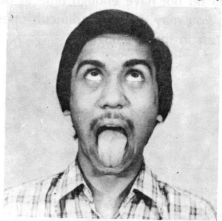

Fig. 8.2

In this position, the facial muscles are stretched. Maintain this position of the face for ten seconds (twenty slow counts). Then relax the facial muscles, withdraw the tongue, shut the mouth and rest the eyes by keeping them lightly closed for twenty seconds.

Repeat the exercise six times. As practice is gained, gradually increase the number of repetitions to ten.

Notes : (1) All facial movements should be non-jerky.

(2) Following the completion of this exercise perform a two-minute palming to rest the eyes.

(3) The Atharva Veda has strongly recommended this exercise to strengthen the vision and eyes.

Gains : (1) The blood supply to various facial and eye muscles increases, producing a feeling of warmth and energy. (2) The vision becomes clearer.

Number two : Eye Pressing

Aim : To render eye-tissues flexible.

Props : None.

Method : Sit comfortably (or in the Vajrasana pose, as advised for exercise number one). Contract firmly the muscles around the eyes (especially those of the eye-lids) to create pressure on the eye-balls (see the photograph below).

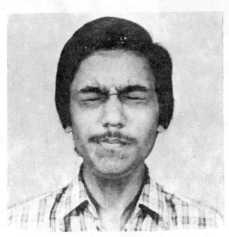

Fig. 8.3

Maintain the contraction for ten slow counts. Finally, let the facial muscles go limp and slack for twenty counts.

Repeat the exercise six times. As practice is gained, gradually increase the number of repetitions to ten.

> **Note :** To rest the eyes following the completion of this exercise, perform palming for two minutes or longer.

Gains : (1) The blood-flow towards the eyes increases. (2) The various eye-tissues (especially the sclera) become elastic and flexible.

Number three : Neck Exercises

Aim : To relax the muscles of the neck and the face and to facilitate the blood-flow towards the eyes.

Props : None.

Method : Sit comfortably on a chair or a small table. Slowly bend the head forward as much as possible (try to touch the chest with the chin). Then bend the head backward as much as possible (see photographs below).

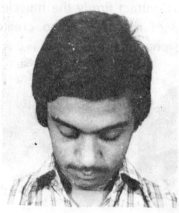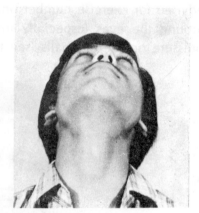

Fig. 8.4

Repeat ten times.

Next, bend the head, as much as possible, towards the right shoulder. Then bend it towards the left shoulder (see photographs on the next page).

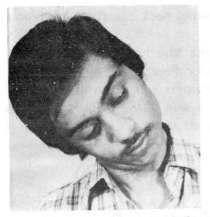 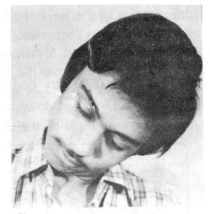

Fig. 8.5

Repeat the action ten times.

Next, turn the head, as much as possible, towards the right. Then turn it towards the left (see photographs below).

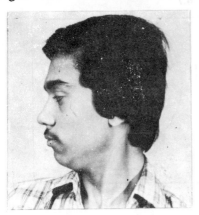 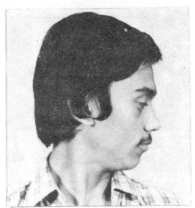

Fig. 8.6

Repeat the action ten times.

Finally, rotate the head in circles twenty times. To avoid giddiness, rotate the head five times in one direction (clockwise), five times in the other direction (anticlockwise) and so on.

> **Note :** In the entire exercise, the head should be moved in a smooth, non-jerky manner.

Gains : (1) The neck and the facial muscles are relaxed.
(2) The arteries supplying nourishment to the eyes lie between

the muscles of the neck. Following neck exercises, the blood-flow to the eyes increases.

Number four : Shirshasana (the head stand)

Aim : To improve the blood-flow to the eyes.

Props : A blanket or a mattress spread on the ground.

Method : Kneel down at a side of the blanket. Interlock the fingers and place the hands on the ground in such a

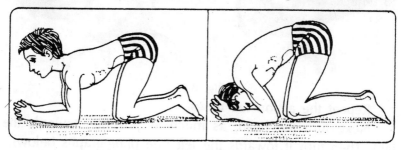

Fig. 8.7

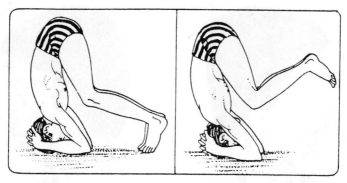

Fig. 8.8

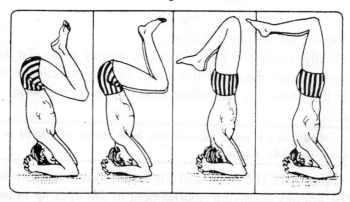

Fig. 8.9

way that the backs of the palms and the elbows remain in contact with the ground. Place the back of the top of the head on the palms. Now raise the trunk and lift the legs off the floor gradually. Finally, step by step, attain a vertical position, with head below and legs at the top. Keep the eyes closed. Maintain this posture for about fifteen seconds. As experience is gained, the time can be increased gradually to about one minute.

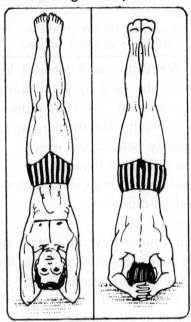

Fig. 8.10

Finally, bring the legs down (step by step, in the reverse order).

It is absolutely necessary to lie down on the ground for a few minutes following Shirshasana.

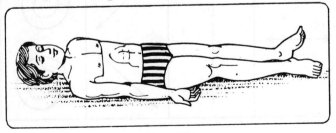

Fig. 8.11

> **Notes :** (1) Shirshasana should be performed with an empty stomach.
>
> (2) Initially, the final position of this asana is difficult to attain. If balancing seems difficult, the person can rest his legs against a wall or some support.
>
> (3) Persons who fail to learn this asana can perform another asana called Sarvangasana (the shoulder stand), to obtain almost similar benefits. The method of performing this asana can be learnt from a good book on yoga.
>
> (4) Upside-down postures like Shirshasana or Sarvangasana are prohibited for persons with high blood pressure.

Gains : (1) Since the head remains low, a lot of extra blood is brought to the eyes by gravitational pull. Thus, the eyes are richly nourished. (2) The asana affects the brain favourably, thus improving the memory and the visualisation-power. This indirectly benefits the eyes.

Number five : Thumb Pursuits

Aim : To exercise the muscles that move the eyes and to develop eye-hand co-ordination.

Props : None.

Method : Sit comfortably on a chair or a table. Extend your hand at an arm's length directly in front of your nose. Make a fist, excluding your thumb. Point your thumb upward so that you can view its nail.

Steadily looking at the thumbnail, move your hand (in as big arcs as possible) in the following directions :

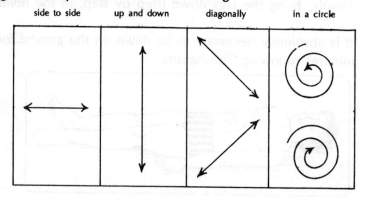

Fig. 8.12

Move your hand ten times in either direction. The movement should be smooth and non-jerky. Try not to move your body or head.

> Note : Following the completion of the exercises, perform palming for two minutes or more.

Gains : (1) The muscles that move the eyes become more flexible and strong. (2) Any eye-strain arising out of an imbalance of these muscles is relieved, since the eyes slowly learn to work in a more co-ordinated manner. (3) Stiffness of the eye-muscles, arising due to prolonged periods of tasks requiring concentration (e.g., typing, proof-reading etc.), is relieved. (4) Eye to hand co-ordination improves.

Number six : Eye Tracking

Aim : To be able to follow a moving object continuously with the eyes.

Props : A small and pointed object like a pencil or a pen.

Method : Sit comfortably on a chair or a table. Hold the pen in your hand, with its tip pointing upwards. Extend the arm. Steadily looking at the pen-tip, move your hand smoothly and rapidly ten times in each of the following directions :

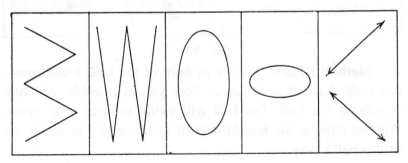

Fig. 8.13

Concentrate on the pen-tip. Do not allow your sight to wander even for a second from the pen-tip. Do not try to keep your head or the body steady.

> Note : After completing the exercise, rest the eyes by performing palming for two minutes or more.

Gain : This exercise develops the ability of the eyes to follow a fast-moving object smoothly and uninterruptedly.

Number seven : Dodge ball

Aim : To develop good co-ordination between the eyes and the body.

Props : A soft ball suspended at about chest height from the ceiling.

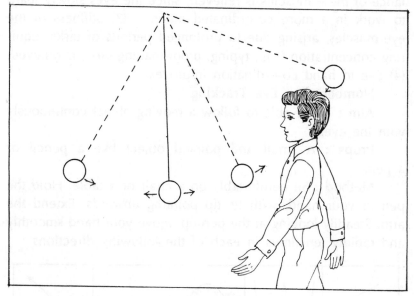

Fig. 8.14

Method : Stand directly in front of the ball. Have some-one hold the ball as far away from you as possible. Ask him to release the ball. The ball will swing towards your chest. Without moving the feet from their positions, try to move out of the ball's way.

When the ball is behind your back, try to judge its speed and position. Continuing to look forward, move your body so that the ball does not hit you on the back-swing.

If you do not have anybody to help you, just move the ball away from you to do the exercise.

Continue the exercise as long as you enjoy it.

Gains : Co-ordination between the eyes and the body develops. Ability to judge accurately the objects in the space also develops.

VISUALISATION EXERCISES

Visualisation exercises serve to relax the various eye muscles, facilitate focus-control and thus improve the eyesight. These exercises utilise imagination to aid the vision. Most of these exercises can be performed not only by persons having visual defects but also by those who desire to keep their eyes and vision strong and efficient. Some of these exercises are, however, specific for specific visual defects.

Number one : Visualising movements associated with breathing

This exercise is the simplest of various visualisation exercises. It can be done at any time, anywhere. It is extremely soothing and relaxes the body and the mind. The eyes, too, get relaxed and eye-strain is relieved.

Aim : To visualise the movements of lungs, the chest and the abdomen during respiration.

Props : None.

Method : Lie down on the floor or sit in a comfortable arm-chair, in a quiet room. Keep your eyes closed. Let all your muscles go limp and slack. Focus your attention on the process and rythm of your breathing. Lungs are like balloons. Imagine them expanding as they get filled with air when you breathe in. To accommodate this expansion, the chest and the abdomen also expand. Visualise these movements mentally. While breathing out, imagine the chest and the abdomen contracting and the lungs deflating.

Continue this visualisation exercise for two to three minutes.

Note : It may take you some time to accomplish this exercise successfully.

Gains : All the muscles of the body, including those of the eyes get relaxed. Relaxation is the key to unstrained and efficient vision.

Number two : Visualising a distant scene

This exercise involves the use of imagination to control (in fact, to release) focusing. Keeping the eyes closed, we 'paint' a distant scene with our mind. We direct our mind's eye to an imaginary far horizon, a distant mountain-top or a ship at the sea. If possible, the scene should be a familiar one, so that the mental image is more accurate and easier to conjure up.

This exercise teaches us to stretch out our gaze, to relax the crystalline lens of our eye and to get used to the feeling of shifting the focus from near to far.

Aim : To visualise a distant scene with the mind's eye.

Props : None

Method : Sit comfortably in a quiet room. Close your eyes. Think of a familiar distant scene. Try to fill in details like colours, textures and weather so that the imagined picture is quite vivid. Observe the horizon. Notice the size, shape and movements of distant objects. Feel the sun warming your eyelids and body. Feel how relaxed your eyes are.

Holding that eye-position, open your eye-lids. The most distant objects around you should be immediately in focus and, therefore, clear, unless your eye-glass prescription is too strong to overcome.

Such imagination of a distant scene for a minute or two and opening the eyes thereafter (with eyeballs still directed at distance) constitutes one cycle. Perform three to five such cycles.

> **Note** : If you are making your child do this exercise, narrate the scene to it : ''Imagine a distant boat in the sea. See how far the ocean stretches; notice how small the boat is. Now watch the boat sailing towards the shore where you are standing. It is approaching very slowly, getting larger and larger in size. Now you can see the sailors standing on its deck. What kind of ship is it ? What is its colour ? Does

it have sails ? Tell me about what you see. Now, send it back out to the sea. Watch it as it gets smaller and smaller."

At this moment, ask your child to open its eyes. Distant objects around it should be immediately in focus and, therefore, quite clear (at least clearer than what they previously were).

Gains : This exercise is especially indicated for near-sighted individuals. Myopes tend to hold their focus too tight. This exercise teaches them to release the focus and experience how it feels when the eye-muscles are relaxed during the distant gaze.

Number three : Visualising distant letters

This exercise is a refined form of visualisation exercise number two. This exercise, too, teaches us to stretch out our gaze and to relax the crystalline lens of our eye.

Aim : To visualise distant letters with the mind's eye.

Props : The distant-vision testing chart provided at the end of this book.

Glasses : Use glasses· only if you cannot read even the first (biggest) letter of the chart from a distance of five feet (i.e., if your visual defect is extremely big).

Method : Hang the chart on the wall at a height of about three feet from the ground. The chart should be well illuminated. Sit on a small table at such a distance from the chart, that the letters of the fourth line can just be read (i.e., the letters of the fifth line cannot be read). Note this distance. Persons with smaller visual defects will be able to sit at a greater distance and those with bigger visual defects at a relatively lesser distance from the chart.

Now direct your gaze at the topmost letter of the chart. Once or twice, move your eyesight along the letter in the same manner as it is written. Now close the eyes and try to visualise the letter with your mind's eye. Strive for a vivid imagination so that the imagined letter is of the same size, texture and colour-intensity, as the actual letter. Thereafter, on opening the eyes, if the letter appears clearer (than it did when you began), you can infer that your imagination was satisfactory.

In a similar manner, imagine all the letters of the second, the third and the fourth lines one after the other. If you have been able to release your focus, relax the crystalline lenses and visualise properly, the letters in the fourth line will be reasonably clear at the end of the exercise (contrast with the fact that they were just legible when you began).

> **Notes :** (1) After completing the exercise, perform palming for two minutes or more.
>
> (2) If there is a considerable difference (in magnitude or nature) in the visual defect of the two eyes, perform the exercise first with one eye and then the other. Note that the distance where you sit will vary for each eye.
>
> (3) As your ability to release the focus and relax the crystalline lens increases and as vision improves, progressively increase the distance from where you do the exercise (keeping visibility of the letters of the fourth line as the criterion).

Gains : This exercise relaxes the crystalline lens of the eye and teaches the release of focus. It is especially useful to myopes.

Number four : Visualisation of the candle-flame

Aim : To visualise the flame of a candle with the mind's eye.

Props : A candle, a dark room (with windows closed).

Glasses : Do not use glasses.

Method : Light the candle in a dark room. Prevent exposure of the candle-flame to air-currents so that it remains stable. The candle-flame shows three distinct colours : the central dark spot around the wick, the bright golden yellow colour surrounding the dark spot (and forming

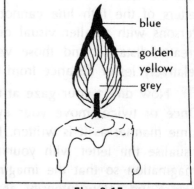

Fig. 8.15

the major part of the flame) and the blue colour at the tip.

Sit about fifteen to eighteen inches away from the candle. Observe the various parts and colours of the flame, for a few seconds.

Close the eyes and visualise the flame with your mind's eye. This is comparatively easier because of the formation of 'after-image'. (After-images are spots of light that temporarily remain on our retina after we look at a bright light. They result from temporary bleaching of the photo-retinal cells. The area on the retina that was activated by the bright light retains that image, while the surrounding areas of the retina remain unbleached and, therefore, seem dark by contrast). Try to make your imagination as vivid as possible, visualising all the three colours. After a few seconds, as the after-image grows indistinct, open your eyes.

Repeat the entire procedure three to five times.

Note : At the end perform palming for two minutes or more.

Gains : This exercise makes us experience how it feels when the muscles of the eyes contract while concentrating on a near object. Therefore, this exercise is especially useful for persons with hypermetropia.

Number five : Visualising near letters

This exercise is an advanced form of visualisation exercise number four. This exercise, too, teaches us to draw in our gaze and focus, the near objects clearly.

Aim : To visualise near letters with the mind's eye.

Props : The letter chart given below.

Glasses : Do not use glasses.

Method : Hold the chart in your hands, at a distance of about fifteen inches from the eyes. The chart should be well illuminated.

Direct your gaze at the topmost letters of the chart. Move your eyesight along the letter in the same manner as it is written. Now close the eyes and try to visualise the letter with your mind's eye. Strive for a vivid imagination so that the imagined letter is of the same size and colour intensity as the actual letter. Thereafter, on opening the eyes, if you find the letter immediately in focus and quite clear, you can infer that your visualisation was satisfactory.

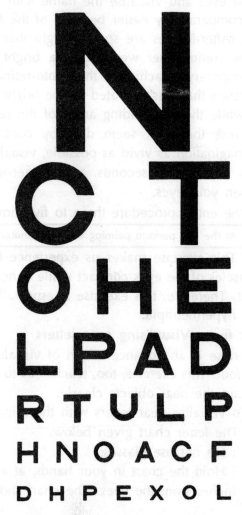

Fig. 8.16

In a similar manner, imagine one after the other, all the letters in the second, the third and the fourth lines.

Note : At the end of the exercise, perform palming for two minutes or more.

Gains : This exercise strengthens the ability to draw in the focus, required while performing near-point tasks and which the hypermetropes are found to lag in.

Number six : Practice on white intersections

Aim : To visualise an increase in whiteness (i.e., clarity) of the intersections of the vertical and horizontal white lines.

Props : The chart given below

Glasses : Do not use glasses.

Method : Hold the chart in your hands, about fifteen inches away from the eyes.

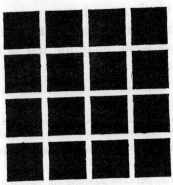

Fig. 8.17

Direct your gaze to the white intersection of the uppermost horizontal and the left vertical white lines. Looking intently at the intersection, blink for three-four times rapidly. If your visualisation has been correct, you will see the intersection whiter than it actually is. On the other hand, if you have not drawn in your focus adequately and have not concentrated, you will see a grey shadow superimposed upon the white intersection.

Similarly, concentrate on the rest of the nine intersections. Repeat the entire procedure two to three times.

Notes : (1) As ability increases, hold the chart closer and closer to the eyes.
(2) In the end, perform palming for two minutes or more.

Gains : Ability to draw in the focus and concentrate on near objects develops. Thus, the exercise is especially useful to hypermetropes and presbyopes.

Number seven : Practice on white lines

Aim : To visualise an increase in whiteness (i.e., clarity) of the empty white spaces (called white lines) between two printed lines.

Props : Any book with snow-white paper and good printing.

Glasses : Do not use glasses.

Method : Hold the book upside down (i.e., inverted), about fifteen inches from your eyes.

Blinking slowly and continuously, move your eyesight slowly along the blank space between any two printed lines. If your visualisation is satisfactory, you should see that part of the white line more white (than the rest of the line) at which your gaze is directed.

Continue the exercise for about two minutes (i.e., about half a page of the book).

> **Note** : (1) As experience is gained and ability to draw in the focus improves, decrease the distance between the book and your eyes gradually.
>
> (2) At the end, perform palming for two minutes or more.

Gains : This exercise is especially useful to presbyopes and hyperopes as it develops the ability to draw the focus inwards.

FOCAL FLEXIBILITY EXERCISES

The ability to shift focus easily and smoothly from near to far (and vice versa) is essential for efficient vision. Developing this ability helps overcome the effects of functional vision problems. An inflexibility of the crystalline lens gives rise to eye-strain and the various symptoms associated with it. The exercises to be described now make our lens more flexible and efficient, allowing us to make full use of our visual potential and prevent or decrease existent visual defects.

Number one : Fingernail pursuit

Aim : To develop the ability to shift focus rapidly by increasing the flexibility of the crystalline lens.

Props : None

Glasses : Do not use glasses.

Method : Hold the index finger of one of your hands near your nose tip. Fix your gaze on the finger-tip. Move your hand away from your nose till your arm is fully stretched. Thereafter, bring the finger back to your nose-tip. Continue looking at the tip of your finger all the time.

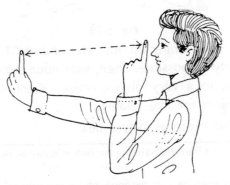

Fig. 8.18

Repeat the exercise twenty times.

Note : At the end, perform palming for two minutes or more.

Gains : The crystalline lenses of the eyes become or remain flexible, an important requisite for quick and accurate focusing.

Number two : Alternate near and far gaze

Aim : To develop the ability to shift focus from far to near and vice versa quickly and accurately, by increasing the flexibility of the crystalline lens.

Props : None

Glasses : Do not use glasses.

Method : Stand near an open window. Hold the index finger of one of your hands stationary near the tip of your nose.

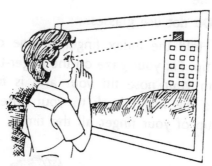

Fig. 8.19

Look at your finger-tip for five counts. Try to see the finger as clearly as possible. Then, shift your gaze, through the open window, to a very distant object. Continue looking at the distant object for five counts.

Repeat the exercise forty times.

> **Notes :** (1) Perform palming for two minutes or more, following the exercise.
>
> (2) This exercise can be done advantageously following a long session of reading or writing (or any other type of near-point work).

Gains : This exercise makes the crystalline lens more flexible and hence enhances our ability to shift focus quickly from near to far (and vice versa).

Number three : Alternate near and far reading

This exercise is an advanced form of focal flexibility exercise number two.

Aim : To render the crystalline lens of the eye more flexible and efficient.

Props : The distant-vision testing chart (provided at the end of this book), the near-vision testing chart (given at the end of this book).

Glasses : Use glasses only if your distant or near vision is too weak.

Method : Hang the distant-vision testing chart on the wall, at a height of about three feet from the ground. Ensure good illumination on this chart. Sit at such a distance from the chart that at least the first four lines can be read.

Hold the near-vision testing chart (pasted on a cardboard for ease in handling) in your hands, about fifteen inches from your eyes.

Direct your gaze to the near chart. For a few seconds, read the smallest letters that are legible. Then shift your gaze to the distant chart. For a few seconds, read the letters of that chart. The procedure described so far constitutes one cycle.

Perform ten such cycles. Note how long it takes to see clearly when you change gaze from one chart to the other.

> **Notes :** (1) At the end, perform palming for two minutes or more.
>
> (2) As your ability and your lenses' flexibility increase, gradually sit further away from the distant chart and hold the near-vision testing chart closer to your eyes.

Gains : The crystalline lens becomes more flexible and efficient.

Number four : Reading at continually changing distance

Aim : To make the crystalline lens more flexible and responsive to subtle changes in the distance of reading material.

Props : A book with good printing.

Glasses : Use glasses only if unavoidable for near-point work.

Method : Hold the book about fifteen inches from your eyes. Start reading.

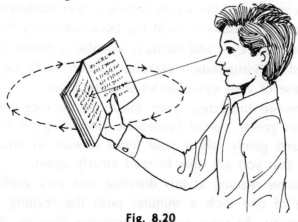

Fig. 8.20

Continuing your reading move the book slowly in small horizontal circles so that the book alternately approaches you and recedes away from you.

Try to maintain clear vision throughout the entire range of the circular motion of the book.

Continue the exercise for about two minutes.

> **Notes :** (1) At the end, perform palming for two minutes or more.
>
> (2) As your ability and your lenses' flexibility increase, move the book faster and in larger circles, trying to maintain clear vision all the time.

Gain : The lens becomes more flexible and the ability to shift focus increases rapidly. This exercise is especially indicated for persons aged around forty.

Number five : Reading out

This exercise is especially indicated for persons with myopia.

Aim : To increase the distance at which reading is possible.

Props : A book with good printing.

Glasses : Do not use glasses.

Method : Sit at a place where the illumination is very good. Hold the book at such a distance from where you can easily read. Continuing reading, push the reading material gradually away from the eyes (at the rate of one inch every thirty seconds) until the vision begins to blur moderately. This is the first blur distance. Hold the book stationary here.

Close your eyes and mentally visualise a distant scene (as described in 'visualisation exercise number two'). Experience the release of your eye-muscles and the focus.

Continue projecting your vision at distance and open your eyes gently. Avoid immediate refocusing on the page. Slowly and gently, allow your focus to ease in towards the page so that you are able to read clearly again.

Resume reading at this distance and very gradually (at the rate of one inch a minute) push the reading material further away. As soon as you encounter blurring of vision, close your eyes repeat the steps of distant visualisation and thereafter drawing in the focus.

Continue to do this, until you can no longer expand the reading distance. Note this distance.

> **Notes** : (1) At. the end, perform palming for two minutes or more.
>
> (2) Incorporate this exercise into your daily activities, i.e., to say, read for at least fifteen minutes at your longest reading distance.

Gains : Myopes hold their focus too tight. This exercise teaches them to release the focus, which in turn ensures that the defect does not progress unchecked.

Number six : Reading in

This exercise is especially indicated for persons with hypermetropia or presbyopia.

Aim : To decrease the distance at which reading is possible.

Props : A book with good printing.

Glasses : Do not use glasses, unless you are a presbyope requiring strong glasses for reading.

Method : Sit at a place where the illumination is very good. Hold the book in your hands, at a distance as far as necessary to establish clear vision.

Gradually, draw the reading material closer to your eyes (approximately one inch every thirty seconds) until the vision just begins to blur. This is the first blur distance. At this moment, stop the movement of the book.

Close your eyes and mentally visualise an object which is closer to your eyes by about five inches, as compared to the book. Strive for vivid imagination.

Continue to hold the focus close and gently open your eyes. Avoid immediate refocusing on the page. Thereafter, slowly release your focus towards the book. The letters should be clearly visible.

Resume reading at this distance and bring the book gradually towards you. As soon as you encounter blurring, close the eyes and repeat the process of visualisation of very near objects and then release of the focus slowly to reach the book.

Continue to do this till you can no longer decrease the reading distance. Note this distance.

> **Notes :** (1) At the end, perform palming for two minutes or more.
>
> (2) For at least fifteen minutes every day, read at the closest possible distance.

Gains : Hyperopes and presbyopes cannot draw in their focus adequately. This exercise teaches them to do so and thereby ensures that the defect does not progress unchecked.

EXERCISES TO OVERCOME MUSCLE-IMBALANCES AND STRENGTHEN FUSION

Refractive errors like myopia, hypermetropia or astigmatism are, many a time, found associated with muscular imbalances (hidden squints) or anomalies of fusion. On the other hand, muscular imbalances can give rise to eye-strain and thus precipitate defects of vision.

The exercises described here are designed to develop accurate fixation with both eyes, teach proper control (tighten or release, as the need be) of focal power and stimulate equal and simultaneous use of the two eyes.

The key to the successful performance of these exercises is relaxation. Use your eyes in a relaxed and not-too-hard manner. This allows information-transmitting nerve circuits from both the eyes to work.

These exercises can be done advantageously even by persons with good sight and strong eyes.

Number one : String exercise

The procedure involved in this exercise has previously been discussed in the chapter on self-assessment. Here we are going to use it for practising fixation, correcting convergence and overcoming suppression. This is a good exercise to demonstrate that each eye forms its own image of an object.

Aim : To achieve correct fixation and simultaneous perception (with two eyes) and to overcome suppression, if any.

Props : A string which is at least fifteen feet long, and three buttons that can be beaded onto the string.

Glasses : Use glasses only if absolutely necessary to obtain clear vision.

Method : Tie one end of the string to a door-knob. Bead the three buttons onto the string in such a way that they lie six

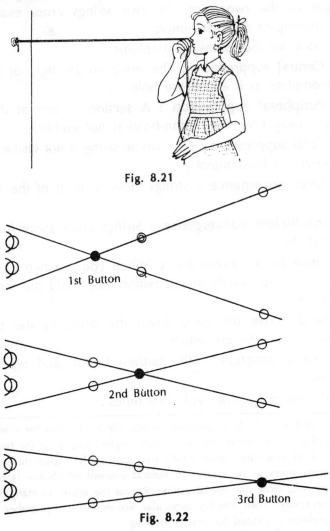

Fig. 8.21

Fig. 8.22

inches, eighteen inches and four feet from the other (i.e., untied) end of the string. Hold the string taut against your nose tip.

Look at the hole in the first (nearest) button. You should see two strings going through the button-hole. If the right eye is closed, the left string seems to disappear; if the left eye is closed, the right string seems to disappear. If you have directed your eyes correctly, and if the brain registers the images of the two eyes, the two strings cross exactly at the opening of the first button.

Look for the following problems :

Central suppression : The string on the right or the left is incomplete as it enters the hole.

Peripheral suppression : A section of one at the two strings (away from the button-hole) is not visible.

Total suppression : One whole string is not visible either constantly or intermittently.

Overconvergence : Strings cross in front of the button-hole.

Insufficient convergence : Strings cross away from the button-hole.

Strive for a relaxed focus. When you see two complete strings crossing exactly at the button-hole, hold the focus for ten counts.

Next, move the gaze down the string to the second button. Repeat the procedure.

Finally, progress to the farthest button and repeat the exercise.

Repeat the entire cycle five times.

Notes : (1) If suppression occurs, close the eyes for a while. Visualise in your mind, the two strings crossing exactly at the button-hole. Then open the eyes and refix your gaze softly. Repeat this action as many times as necessary. To remind yourself which eye is being suppressed, close one eye at a time. Repeat the action as many times as necessary. Then employ binocular vision softly. Remember that suppression is caused by intense viewing.

(2) If over-convergence occurs, close your eyes and visualise a distant scene, thereby stretching your gaze. Then reopen your eyes. Keep the gaze extended. Draw it in very slowly until the strings cross at the hole.

(3) If under-convergence occurs, close your eyes and visualise a very near object (say your nose-tip). Feel your eyes pulling in. Then reopen your eyes. Release the focus slowly until the strings cross at the hole.

(4) At the end of the exercise, perform palming for two minutes or more.

(5) As you gain practice and experience, alter the positions of the buttons to encounter new challenges :

Period	Distance of the three buttons from the nose-tip		
First week	ten inches	eighteen inches	four feet
Second week	eight inches	fourteen inches	eight feet
Third week	six inches	twelve inches	twelve feet
Fourth week	four inches	ten inches	fifteen feet

Gain : This exercise necessitates seeing with both the eyes together and hence overcomes suppression.

Number two : The 'X' card

Aim : To control convergence of the two eyes and to stimulate simultaneous perception.

Props : An 'X' card of the size 3" x 5", the sample of which has been given below.

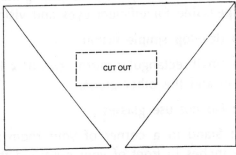

Fig. 8.23

Glasses : Use glasses only if absolutely necessary for clear vision.

Method : Draw an 'X' card on a piece of cardboard and cut out the portions indicated.

Hold the card in front of your eyes, six inches from the nose. Shift your gaze through the top opening of the card to a distant object. The two inclined lines should cross each other to form the figure of X, in the middle of the card.

Correctly adjust your focus so that the top and the bottom arms of 'X' are of the same length.

Hold the 'X' in view for five counts. Then close the eyes and relax.

Complete ten such cycles.

> Notes : (1) At the end, perform palming for two minutes or more.
> (2) The distance of the 'X' card from the eyes should be varied thus :
> First week – six inches
> Second week – ten inches
> Third week – fourteen inches
> Fourth week – as far away from eyes as possible.

Gain : This procedure exercises the convergence and compels us to view with both the eyes together.

Number three : Simple fusion

The two images of an object, formed in our two eyes are fused into one by the brain. Therefore, we do not see double. Good fusion is like an insurance against squint, i.e., to say, it prevents a latent squint (if any) from becoming manifest. Good fusion is indispensable for efficient eyes and vision.

Aim : To develop simple fusion.

Props : A small rectangular mirror, two 8" x 10" sheets of paper – one red and the other green.

Glasses : Do not use glasses.

Method : Stand in a corner of your room so that one wall is twenty inches in front of your eyes and the side wall is twenty inches from your ear.

Stick the red paper on the wall in front of your eyes at about eye-level. Stick the green paper on the side-wall opposite your ear.

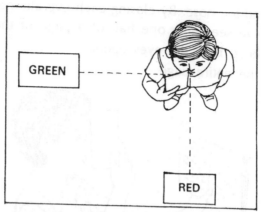

Fig. 8.24

Take the mirror and place it against your nose so that you can look into the mirror with the eye nearest to the side-wall and see the green paper reflected in the mirror. The other eye sees the red paper lying straight ahead.

Adjust the mirror gently so that the red and the green papers become superimposed. Try to see an equal mixture of colours for ten counts. Then close your eyes and relax for a while.

Complete five such cycles.

Repeat the exercise in a different corner of your room so that you have to keep the mirror in front of the other eye.

Note : At the end, perform palming for two minutes or more.

Gain : This exercise helps to overcome suppression and facilitate fusion.

Number four : Reading with a card interposed between the two eyes

Aim : To strengthen fusion.

Props : A big-sized book, a 3" x 6" card.

Glasses : Use glasses only if absolutely necessar clear near vision.

Method : Hold the book about twelve eyes. Hold the card vertically between forehead and the nose. By closing each eye alternately, ensure that each eye sees only one half of a page of the book.

Now keep both the eyes open.

Read the entire page.

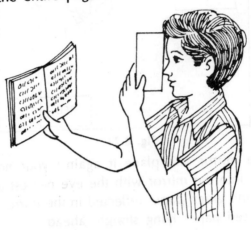

Fig. 8.25

Note : At the end, perform palming for two minutes or more.

Gain : This exercise stimulates simultaneous vision with the two eyes and strengthens fusion.

Number five : Two coins fusion

Aim : To strengthen fusion.

Props : Two identical coins, a pencil.

Glasses : Use glasses only if absolutely necessary for clear vision.

Method : Place the coins on a table, about two inches apart.

The coins should have the same picture and face the same direction.

Sit comfortably in front of the coins. Keep the pencil on ⌐ table with its tip resting on the table between the coins. ⌐ncentrate on the tip of the pencil. Out of the corner of ⌐ aware of the coins.

⌐ the pencil towards your nose, continuing to

As you bring the pencil off the table by

about eight inches, you should notice through your peripheral vision that, at first, the coins double (to four coins) and then the central coins finally merge into one. Thus, you now see three coins : the original left one, the merged one and the original right one.

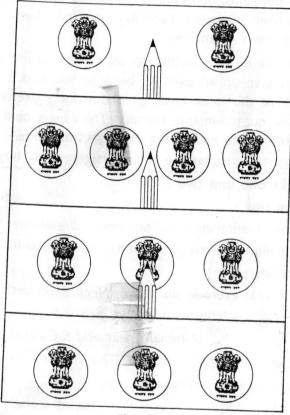

Fig. 8.26

After keeping the fused image in view for 10 counts, close the eyes and relax for a while.

Repeat the cycle five times.

Note : At the end, perform palming for two minutes or more.

Gain : The ability to fuse the two images of the two retinae improves

9. VISION TRAINING PROGRAMMES

This chapter presents basic vision training programmes for errors of refraction like myopia, hypermetropia, presbyopia, astigmatism and amblyopia. Besides these, supplementary schedules for the treatment of eye-problems like suppression, convergence problems, muscular imbalances and latent squint have also been suggested. Each day's routine takes about half to three quarters of an hour.

It would be worthwhile to state here again that you should not give up an exercise because you find it difficult; stick to it. At the same time, go about doing exercises in a relaxed and not-too-intense manner. The eyes should not feel unduly tired at the end of the exercise-programme.

Suggested programme for nearsightedness (myopia)

Weeks one and two :

	Page No.
Warm ups :	
1. Visualisation exercise no. one *(Breathing)*	75
2. General exercise no. seven *(Dodge ball)*	74
Exercises :	
1. General exercise no. three *(Neck exercises)*	68
2. Focal flexibility exercise no. two *(Alternate near and far gaze)*	83
3. General exercise no. five *(Thumb pursuits)*	72
4. Visualisation exercise no. two *(Distant scene)*	76
5. General exercise no. two *(Eye pressing)*	67

Weeks three and four :

	Page No.
Warm ups :	
1. Visualisation exercise no. one *(Breathing)*	75
2. General exercise no. three *(Neck exercises)*	68

Exercises :

1. Focal flexibility exercise no. one   82
                                   (Fingernail pursuit)

2. Visualisation exercise no. three (Distant letters)   77

3. Focal flexibility exercise no. three
                      (Alternate near and far reading)   84

4. General exercise no. two   (Eye pressing)   67

5. Focal flexibility exercise no. five
                                    (Reading out)   86

Suggested programme for farsightedness (hypermetropia)

Weeks one and two :

Warm ups :   Page No.

1. Visualisation exercise no. one   (Breathing)   75

2. General exercise no. four   (Shirshasana)   70

Exercises :

1. General exercise no. three
                                  (Neck exercises)   68

2. Focal flexibility exercises no. two
                      (Alternate near and far gaze)   83

3. General exercise no. one   (Sinhasana)   66

4. Visualisation exercise no. four
                                  (Candle-flame)   78

5. General exercise no. five (Thumb pursuits)   72

Weeks three and four

Warm ups :   Page No.

1. Visualisation exercise no. one   (Breathing)   75

2. General exercise no. three
                                  (Neck exercises)   68

Exercises :

1. Focal flexibility exercise no. one
                                  (Fingernail pursuit)   82

2. General exercise no. five *(Thumb pursuits)* — 72

3. Focal flexibility exercise no. three
   (Alternate near and far reading) — 84

4. Visualisation exercise no. five
   (Near letters) — 79

5. Focal flexibility exercise no. six
   (Reading in) — 87

Suggested programme for presbyopia

Weeks one and two :

Warm ups :   Page No.

1. Visualisation exercise no. one   *(Breathing)* — 75

2. General exercise no. four   *(Shirshasana)* — 70

Exercises :

1. General exercise no. three
   (Neck exercises) — 68

2. Visualisation exercise no. six
   (White intersections) — 80

3. Focal flexibility exercise no. two
   (Alternate near and far gaze) — 83

4. General exercise no. one   *(Sinhasana)* — 66

5. Visualisation exercise no. four
   (Candle-flame) — 78

Weeks three and four :

Warm ups :   Page No.

1. Visualisation exercise no. one *(Breathing)* — 75

2. General exercise no. three *(Neck exercises)* — 68

Exercises :

1. Focal flexibility exercise no. three
   (Alternate near and far reading) — 84

2. General exercise no. five *(Thumb pursuits)* — 72

3. Focal flexibility-exercise no. four
                (*Reading at changing distances*) $\boxed{85}$
4. Visualisation exercise no. seven
                              (*White lines*) $\boxed{82}$
5. Focal flexibility exercise no. six
                              (*Reading in*) $\boxed{87}$

Suggested programme for astigmatism

Weeks one and two :

Warm ups :   **Page No.**

1. Visualisation exerci,e no. one   (*Breathing*) $\boxed{75}$

2. General exercise no. seven   (*Dodge ball*) $\boxed{74}$

Exercises :

1. General exercise no. three (*Neck exercises*) $\boxed{68}$
2. Focal flexibility exercise no. two
                (*Alternate near and far gaze*) $\boxed{83}$

3. General exercise no. two   (*Eye pressing*) $\boxed{67}$
4. Visualisation exercise no. two
                              (*Distant scene*) $\boxed{76}$

5. General exercise no. five (*Thumb pursuits*) $\boxed{72}$

Weeks three and four :

Warm ups :   **Page No.**

1. Visualisation exercise no. one   (*Breathing*) $\boxed{75}$

2. General exercise no. three (*Neck exercises*) $\boxed{68}$

Exercises :

1. General exercise no. one   (*Sinhasana*) $\boxed{66}$
2. Visualisation exercise no. two
                              (*Distant scene*) $\boxed{76}$

3. General exercise no. two   (*Eye pressing*) $\boxed{67}$

4. Focal flexibility exercise no. three
                (*Alternate near and far reading*) $\boxed{84}$

5. General exercise no. five (*Thumb pursuits*) $\boxed{72}$

Suggested programme for lazy eye (amblyopia)

Binocular amblyopia (laziness of both eyes) is usually the result of high refractive errors not corrected (with glasses) in time. Therefore, the first part of the treatment would consist of getting glasses of appropriate powers. Thereafter, the exercise programme will depend upon whether you have myopia or hypermetropia.

Amblyopia (laziness) of only one eye may be the result of either uncorrected uniocular high refractive error or long-standing squint of the affected eye. Professional eye-examination is necessary to determine the cause and severity of the problem. Thereafter, the most important part of the treatment consists of occluding (i.e., keeping covered) the vision of the good eye for as long as possible during the day. Thus, the lazy eye is compelled to work and see and therefore, improves rapidly. Besides, an exercise programme as applicable for myopia or hypermetropia or squint, depending upon the cause, should be employed.

It was once believed that amblyopia of adults cannot be helped much. But now that view is being discared because it has been seen that even old case of amblyopia respond favourably to occlusion and exercises. Better late than never !

Supplemental programmes for problems like suppression, convergence problems or muscular imbalances

Suggested programme for suppression :   Page No.

1. String exercise   88
2. Simple fusion exercise   92
3. Reading with a card interposed between the two eyes   93

Suggested programme for convergence problems : Page No.

1. Focal flexibility exercise no. one
                      (Fingernail pursuit)   82
2. String exercise   88
3. The 'X' card exercise   91
4. Two coin fusion exercise   94

It should be noted that a refractive error (e.g., myopia) and a muscular problem (e.g., convergence insufficiency or exophoria) may co-exist in a person. Such a person will have to do exercises simultaneously to correct both types of defects.

---

10. DECREASE THE DEPENDENCE ON GLASSES

One purpose of this book is to create a society in which every second or third person is not required to use glasses all the time. Today, most spectacle wearers are seen to have become so much dependent upon glasses that they feel helpless without them and reach for them the first thing in the morning. The glasses then part company with the bridge of the nose and ears only at night.

It is known that concentrated viewing tenses the eye muscles and the crystalline lens. This may force a person's eyes to work very hard without realising it. When glasses are used, this intense concentration develops more readily since images are clearer and frames act like blinders to limit peripheral awareness. Again, glasses make it unnecessary for the eyes to work on their own. Since the glasses substitute their power for the natural power of the eyes, innate visual abilities diminish through disuse. It is a common experience that following prolonged use of glasses, unaided vision (vision without glasses) deteriorates; a person who could previously read three or four lines of the chart without glasses can later read only one or two (in spite of the fact that the spectacle numbers have not gone up).

Vision is a dynamic process. Its sharpness undergoes small changes during the day. Under favourable conditions or in the absence of strain, the vision is sharper. However, its sharpness declines if eyes are strained.

Along with the sharpness of vision, the error of refraction (i.e., the visual defect) also undergoes small changes. This is a proven fact. If causative factors are not at work, a visual defect may decrease spontaneously, partially or totally. For example, excessive and concentrated near-point work is the chief cause of nearsightedness or myopia. If one keeps away from reading or writing for a considerable length of time, myopia may decrease. A number of studies have shown that the percentage of myopia in youngsters is greater during the school year than at the end of a long vacation, a time of few books and long hours outdoors. Yet few doctors take this into consideration while prescribing glasses at the end of the school year, unaware that the condition might improve during the vacation.

To see clearly through a particular glass, the eye has to continuously maintain the visual defect, which is otherwise liable to small changes. In other words, once glasses are used, the eye stays in its myopic state until it becomes permanently nearsighted.

Glasses are only a palliative measure in the treatment of visual defects. They do not reach the root of the problem. They may enable a person to get instant clear vision. But they do not consider the root causes of visual defects and do nothing to check their progress. The popularity that glasses enjoy today is solely because of our passive approach to our visual problems. We expect everything to be done to us, to our eyes; we are not ready to take pains ourselves. The fast life today has snatched away zeal and patience from our minds. When asked to take care of their eyes or to undergo visual training, people frequently say they just do not have time ! But it should be well understood that the less time you give to your eyes today, the more you will have to give later in your life.

This is not to say that glasses are useless. Indeed they might be indispensable for many persons. But they should not form the sole treatment for visual defects. Visual training is of much greater importance.

In myopia, the distant vision is below normal. A myopic child complains that he cannot see the writing on the blackboard. The teacher moves him to the front of the classroom and sends home a note that he should be seen by an eye doctor. He is examined and indeed, distant images are unclear. He is prescribed glasses to enable him to see clearly at distance. No consideration is given to what is causing this problem. In effect, the youngster has been handed a crutch. Glasses do not attempt to help the eyes out of the trouble they have got into, with the hours of reading stress; they merely enforce the abnormal focussing.

Now the child has glasses which help him to see the writing on the blackboard from the back row; but what happens when he shifts his focus back to the book right in front of him ? He had been recommended glasses for 'constant use'. Therefore he continues to do near work with distant glasses. Thus, the eyesight continues to deteriorate, the myopia progressively worsens and the glasses grow thicker. In short, the trend to recommend glasses for constant use is not correct.

When a person is undergoing visual training, constant use of glasses may hinder improvement. Obviously, glasses allow clear vision only if the eyes maintain that much defect continuously, which the glasses intend to correct.

Therefore, doing away with glasses whenever possible is a key step to successful visual training. Albeit, one should be on a constant lookout to avoid eye-strain, by keeping the eyes relaxed. Practical hints about what to do and what not to do when not using glasses have been presented at the end of this chapter.

Certain points about coloured or tinted glasses, too, call for elucidation. Abundant research has clearly shown that all the seven colours of the spectrum are essential for the health of the body and the eyes. If a particular colour is not allowed to enter the eyes for long, a variety of problems may arise. Goggles and tinted glasses do precisely the same thing : Pink glasses completely absorb blue rays and blue glasses completely absorb pink rays and prevent them from entering the eyes.

Albeit special circumstances or special sports (e.g., mountaineering or water-skiing) may demand the use of coloured glasses. But their prolonged use for the sake of fashion or to keep away the sun, is a crime. The use of photochromatic lenses which automatically change from light to dark or vice versa in response to light-intensity is similarly undesirable. The pupil of our eye itself has the ability to contract or expand and thereby control the amount of light entering our eye. To snatch away this adaptation response to light from the pupils and hand over the job to coloured or photochromatic glasses is like using crutches when you have strong legs. With time, the muscles controlling the size of the pupil will become weak.

In short, it can be said that passing some time of the day without glasses is an extremely important step for every person who wishes to prevent further deterioration of his visual defect or who wants to lessen the existing defect.

Do's and Don'ts while not using glasses :

(1) Keep the eyes relaxed. Don't strain your eyes or shut them partially in an effort to make things clearer. This defeats the purpose. Accept the blur. In a short period, the brain will learn to interpret the blurred images correctly.

(2) Close the eyes frequently. This breaks the impulse to strain or focus.

(3) Concentrate on other senses. When going without glasses, rely as much on hearing, touch and smell, as you do on vision.

(4) View the entire scene. Do not concentrate on individual objects or details.

(5) View defensively, not offensively. Be aware of general movements and changes all around.

(6) Shortsighted persons can remove their glasses when they don't need to see at distance, e.g., while reading, writing or conversing. On the other hand, hyperopes (longsighted persons) and presbyopes require glasses especially when they are doing near work. At other times, they can take off their glasses.

(7) Do not listen to your friends' comments that you do not look good without glasses. Your eyes and sight are more important than their opinions or your appearance.

Schedule for 'time without glasses' :

The amount of time you can go without glasses depends on how strong your glass-prescription is. The following chart is a general guide :

(1) Upto + or − 2.00 diopters (numbers) − the more time spent without glasses, the better.

(2) From + or − 2.00 to 6.00 diopters (numbers) − go without glasses for one to three hours a days.

(3) Above + or − 6 diopters (numbers) − go without glasses for 30 to 90 minutes a day.

These guidelines are minimums. As you gain in experience and get accustomed, gradually increase the time without glasses. If you can eat your meals, talk on the phone or travel by public transport without glasses, do it. There is no way to overestimate the value of 'time without glasses'. It breaks our physical and physiological dependence on glasses. It teaches relaxed viewing and enhances our natural visual abilities.

In short, time without glasses is the simplest yet one of the most important and effective of various visual training procedures. It can be integrated into daily activities without any inconvenience. If it becomes a habit, there will be real improvement in the strength of your eyes and clarity of your sight without glasses. Just remember to keep the eyes relaxed. Never strain them. If headaches and eye-fatigue occur when not using glasses, you are trying to overcome the blur instead of accepting it.

11. MAINTENANCE OF IMPROVEMENT

This book recommends a four-week vision-training programme to improve the eye-sight and increase the efficiency of eyes. However, persons with a large (or progressive) visual defect or severe amblyopia can prolong the training to their advantage. In fact, the exercises can be continued indefinitely by incorporating them as part of the daily routine.

After you have improved your eyesight as much as possible, you would like to keep it so or preserve it. Generally, performing 'maintenance exercises' once a week would prove adequate. They can, however, be undertaken more or less frequently, as per individual needs.

If at any time you feel your eye-efficiency or visual sharpness slipping, you can even go back to 'week one' of the original training programme.

Caring for your eyes is one of your most important and life-long responsibilities. Therefore, repeating the entire four-week programme every six months or an year would be desirable.

General guidelines regarding maintenance :

(1) Select any five or six exercises of your liking and requirement.

(2) Change the distance (at which an exercise is performed) or the number of repetitions of exercises constantly so as to preserve interest and encounter a new challenge.

(3) Incorporate the principle of visual training into your daily activities i.e., cultivate them as habits.

● Always be aware of the nature of your visual style and look for specific circumstances to improve it or make it more balanced. For example, during spare time a person with a fixated-central visual style should resist the temptation to read a magazine or a comic-book and instead go for an outing.

● Whenever possible (or following work which has required you to look concentratedly at a particular distance for a long time continuously) go through focal flexibility routines. If you have spare time, practise focal shifts from far to near and vice versa.

● Maintain good eye-hygiene.

● Insist on very good lighting while performing a visual task.

● Do not unduly tire your eyes.

(4) Make 'time without glasses' a regular part of your daily routine. Albeit, it is necessary to keep the eyes relaxed and fully open when not wearing glasses. Making undue efforts to see clearly while not wearing glasses is self-defeating and invites eye-strain.

(5) At least once a year, repeat the entire four-week programme. Remember that eye and vision-care is a lifetime commitment.

(6) Get your eyes and vision examined by an expert at regular intervals, say every six months. Insist on a thorough examination. Remember that good vision is much more than mere reading of all the letters of the chart; it involves a whole spectrum of skills : How well can you use both eyes together ? How well or accurately can you see objects in space ? Can you shift focus from far to near objects (or vice versa) quickly and easily ? Do your eyes converge sufficiently ? Do your eye-muscles work in a balanced manner etc.

(7) Periodically (say every fortnight or a month), assess your distant and near visual acuity as well as eye-efficiency and record the findings on a special card. This will give you an early clue of a change, if any.

12. PREVENTION OF VISUAL DEFECTS

Though this book is primarily meant for persons with developing or existing visual defects, a brief description of ways and means to prevent visual defects will not be out of place. After all, prevention is better than cure.

Those blessed with a good eye-sight can employ vision training to keep their eyes strong and exploit their potential to the utmost.

The following are prime candidates for this approach :

(1) All students who have to engage their eyes in near-point work for prolonged periods.

(2) All persons who have visually demanding jobs, e.g., scholars, teachers, accountants, watch-repairers, diamond assorters, computer personnel, typists, stenographers, clerks etc.

(3) All adults at around the age of forty (when presbyopia usually starts developing).

(4) All children one or both of whose parents have visual defects.

(5) All children who are detected to lean too much towards either fixated-central or scanning peripheral visual style.

Suggested Approach :

(1) Gain knowledge about the correct use of the eyes. Correct yourself if you have been using your eyes in an incorrect manner.

(2) Cultivate such habits as have been proved good for the eyes and the eyesight.

(3) Learn and employ the various methods suggested to rest and refresh tired eyes.

(4) Try to keep your visual style balanced. If you have been fixated-central so far, take a greater interest in outdoor and social activities and refrain from reading unessential books, periodicals or comics. If you have been scanning-peripheral so far, take a greater interest in books and details.

(5) Regular treatment of eyes with appropriate magnets and stimulation of specific acupressure points, too, can keep visual defects at bay. Details have been presented in chapter 14.

(6) Perform a general eye-exercise, a visualisation exercise, a focal flexibility exercise and an exercise to enhance the balance of eye-muscles at least once a week.

(7) Get your eyes and the vision thoroughly examined by a competent professional at least once a year. Remember that merely reading all the letters of the 6/6 (or 20/20) line of the distant chart is not a proof of good vision. Good vision also includes the ability to change focus from near to far objects (and vice versa) easily, to use both eyes in a co-ordinated and harmonious manner etc. Remember that a person could be reading all the letters of the chart and yet could be suffering from a host of visual disorders which affect his outlook and endurance.

13. NUTRITION AND VISION

Very few amongst us are aware of the relation between nutrition and vision. Indeed even the most elite would be able to say no more than 'carrots are good for the eyes'.

Although research demonstrating the importance of vitamins and minerals has been available for many years, it has not been widely circulated or heeded; those who preached the message of nutrition were thought to be alarmists or food faddists. Except for making the general recommendation that one should eat a balanced meal, traditional medicine has relegated nutrition to a back seat.

Today, however, biochemical research has piled up so much data that the connection between good vision and nutrition can no longer be ignored. As a part of a total approach to vision improvement, we present here some of the current data highlighting the relationship of vitamins and minerals to the eyes.

Vitamin A : How often have we heard people say they do not like driving at night because they have trouble seeing ? Or that the glare from the oncoming car 'blinds' them ? Or that driving in the dusky light of sunset is quite bothersome ? They may be deficient in vitamin A. According to one estimate, approximately 20 per cent of the population have this deficiency. So high a figure may be due to one condition of modern life which is difficult to avoid : spending long hours under harsh, glaring lights, which apparently uses up vitamin A at an accelerated rate. So do polluted air, watching a lot of television and keeping awake till late in the night.

Other early symptoms of vitamin A deficiency include burning, itching and inflamed eyes, a feeling that one has sand in the eyes. The condition is called conjunctivitis.

If the vitamin A deficiency is allowed to progress unchecked, the condition of the eyes worsens. Severe deficiency of this vitamin is characterised by extremely dry eyes (xerosis) and night-blindness. Finally, the cornea becomes soft and literally melts (keratomalacia), resulting in permanent blindness. As a matter of fact, vitamin A deficiency is the main cause of blindness in rural India.

Cod liver oil, halibut liver oil, milk, eggs and butter are good sources of vitamin A.

Carrots, mangoes, papaya, cabbage, karelas and green leafy vegetables like coriander, amaranth (tandalja), tulsi, spinach (palakh), mint (phudina), fenugreek (methi), and drumstick leaves contain a substance called carotene, from which the body can make its own vitamin A.

This carotene, present in vegetables and fruits, is extremely sensitive to the atmospheric oxygen. Within twenty minutes of peeling, cutting or scraping vegetables, most of the vitamin A is lost due to oxygenation. Fruits and vegetables should, therefore, be consumed immediately after cutting or peeling them.

Vitamin B Complex : As the name suggests, this is a family of vitamins comprising of such members as B_1, B_2, B_6, B_{12}, B_{15} etc.

If you cannot stand being outdoors in the sunlight even when it is not too bright-without dark sunglasses, a lack of B vitamins could be the culprit. Watery eyes, chronic eye fatigue, light sensitivity, pain behind the eyeball, burning, bloodshot eyes, twilight blindness and seeing just a part of the page or having dark spots in the field of vision may be related to a lack of one or more of the B vitamins and not just insufficiency of vitamin A. If the deficiency is severe, bits of mucous may collect at the base of eyelashes and during sleep the outer corners of the eyes may develop cracks.

As few as 5 mg. of vitamin B_2 has been found to alleviate these symptoms. Evidence suggesting that deficiency of vitamin B_2 may contribute to the development of cataract is piling up. In our country, where millions live on meagre meals containing negligible amounts of vitamins, cataract is common and appears early in life.

At the University of Georgia, 47 persons with a variety of visual problems, including those mentioned above, were given 15 mg. of vitamin B_2 daily. Some of them reported improvement within a day. Six had cataract and after nine months all were reabsorbed; when vitamin B_2 was withdrawn, cataract returned until treatment was resumed. In Russia, too, vitamin B_{15} in combination with vitamins A and E is reported to have produced dramatic results in the treatment of cataract and glaucoma.

Deficiency of vitamin B_{12} may lead to a swelling of the optic nerve, resulting in considerable loss of vision. Difficulty in discerning between red and green colours could also be a consequence of vitamin B_{12} deficiency. Glasses are of no help to such persons.

Our undesirable, and many a time harmful diet has dramatically raised the requirements of B vitamins in our body. Excessive consumption of refined sugar, tea, coffee, cold drinks, tobacco and alcohol deplete the stores of B vitamins in our body.

Liver, eggs, whole cereals, dry fruits and sunflower seeds are good sources of B vitamins. The small amounts of these vitamins present in green vegetables and fruits are destroyed by storing or cooking.

Vitamin C : 'Vitamin C and common cold', a slim book by the Nobel laureate Dr. Linus Pauling, caused ripples in the medical world by claiming that mega-doses of vitamin C not only help to prevent cold and other infections, but also hasten their departure.

Vitamin C is the substance which carries hydrogen to all the cells of our body. Working. with white blood corpuscles, vitamin C fights disease-causing micro-organisms. It is an ingredient which the body uses to manufacture collagen, the binding substance that holds cells and bones together. Since the health of our eyes is closely linked with our general health, it is understandable that adequate vitamin C may be crucial for our eyes.

The healthy lens of the eye is rich in vitamin C, while a diseased lens contains little or none. Glaucoma and cataracts are accompanied by very low levels of vitamin C in the lens, which apparently relates to the fact that old people, who are susceptible to these ailments, are usually found to be efficient in vitamin C.

There is some evidence that vitamin C may be effective in treating glaucoma, a dreadful condition in which the pressure of the fluid inside the eye rise abnormally. In an experiment at the University of Rome, doctors prescribed large doses of vitamin C to patients with severe glaucoma. There was a rapid and significant drop in intra-ocular pressure, with the lowest pressure in the eye when the level of vitamin C in the bloodstream was the highest.

Other researchers have found that large amounts of vitamin C may possibly prevent cataract in diabetics, who are unusually prone to it. A British study reports that healing of corneal ulcers appears to be hastened by taking 1500 mg. of vitamin C daily.

Citrus fruits like lemons, sweet lemons, oranges, amlas, tomatoes, raspberries and papaya are good sources of vitamin C. Vegetables, too, contain it in small amounts.

Vitamin C is easily destroyed by heat and long storage. Therefore, fruits and vegetables should be consumed raw and fresh. If cooking is a must, the water used for cooking or boiling vegetables should not be discarded; it may contain some vitamin C.

Tobacco, mental tension, antibiotic drugs and hormonal drugs deplete or destroy vitamin C present in our body. Smoking just one cigarette destroys about 25 mg. of this useful vitamin.

Vitamin D and Calcium : Although a layman considers vitamin A as the most essential for the eyes, Dr. Arthur Knapp, a New York ophthalmologist gives more importance to vitamin D. Dr. Knapp has treated a number of eye ailments, including myopia successfully, with vitamin D and Calcium. In some cases, the sharpness of vision was more than doubled in a short time. The reports of Dr. Knapp's experiments have appeared in a number of medical magazines, including the Journal of the International Academy of Preventive Medicine.

In an experiment, such patients whose myopia was increasing rapidly were given vitamin D and Calcium. Over fifty per cent showed a change for the better, some remained the same in contrast to the further deterioration that was expected and a full third showed an actual reduction in myopia.

In trials at Columbia's College of Physicians and Surgeons, animals fed diets deficient in vitamin D and Calcium developed a wide range of eye problems.

Apart from myopia, Dr. Knapp has also tried vitamin D and Calcium on humans suffering from several other eye-ailments : keratoconus (a protruding, cone-shaped cornea), cataract, retinitis pigmentosa (a degenerative disease of the retina which leads to night-blindness) and glaucoma. There was a significant improvement in a large percentage of cases. Vitamin D and Calcium go together. In fact, vitamin D is needed for the proper absorption of Calcium, which gives us strong bones and muscles, the eye muscles included. Several studies show that the myopic child is frequently deficient in Calcium.

The vitamin D and Calcium combination seems to dehydrate the fibrous coat of the eyeball. If this coat is waterlogged, it is susceptible to the pressure of the fluid within the eye and stretches into the elongated shape of a nearsighted eye. Due to dehydration of the fibrous coat, the eyeball actually shrinks back to the more normal shape, thereby reducing myopia.

Another researcher, Dr. Hunter Turner, also blames a build up of water pressure in the eye as a prime factor leading to nearsightedness. A high consumption of carbonated soft drinks results in waterlogging inside the body-tissues, including those of the eyeball.

Sunshine is the best natural source of vitamin D. Cod liver (or halibut liver) oil, milk, eggs and butter are some of the other sources.

Milk, green leafy vegetables, beetroot, figs, grapes, bajri (millets), til and black gram (udad) are good sources of Calcium.

Vitamin E : Vitamin E has been credited with doing just about everything : dissolve blood clots, promote the healing of wounds and reducing scars, improve blood-circulation, retard ageing of the cells, keep the heart in good working condition and maintain fertility.

The benefits of vitamin E naturally extend to the eyes. In tests with animals, its lack in the diet caused clouding of the cornea, cataract and other abnormalities of the lens and the retina. It has been shown to be effective in treating numerous eye diseases. In a study undertaken in Italy on 400 patients, uniformly good results were obtained for a variety of eye ailments; in some cases marked visual improvement was noted.

Vitamin E has been shown to enable new blood vessels to form. This may be at least partly responsible for the fact that it appears to be extremely helpful in arresting or even reversing the degenerative changes in the eyes which normally come with old age. In another Italian study, patients over forty years old were given vitamin E, and their presbyopia was reduced to the point where they could once again read without glasses.

Two French doctors working more than two decades ago were able to halt the progress of myopia among young patients by giving them 50-100 mg. of vitamin E daily. Vitamin E has a celubrious effect on the connective tissue or collagen. The doctors proposed that when the collagen fibres of the eyes lose their elasticity, they cannot give the support needed to keep the eye from assuming an abnormal shape if other factors, such as too much near-point work, are putting a stress on the eye. Vitamin E restores elasticity and strength to collagen fibres.

Green leafy vegetables and wheat bran are rich sources of vitamin E.

Protein : We all know that protein in necessary for strength and vitality. It is quite important for the eyes, too. Almost twenty years ago, a British study found a strong relationship between the progress of myopia in children and the amount of protein in the diet.

Half of the children in the experimental group had their diet altered so that ten per cent of their normal calorific intake consisted of animal or vegetable protein; the other half was given no dietary advice. Some of the children over 12 years old in the special diet group showed a definite arrest of myopia. In others, the condition actually reversed itself to some degree. For children under 12 years, the results were less spectacular but still encouraging : while their eyesight continued to deteriorate, the rate of change was slowed down to two-thirds. Those who consumed the most protein showed the least progress of myopia.

Sugar : If nutritionists were asked to name the scourge of the western diet, most of them would put sugar at the top of the list. In recent years, refined sugar has been blamed for everything from dandruff to diabetes. Diabetes is often accompanied by cataract.

Refined sugar, while being processed inside the body, uses up huge quantities of vitamins and minerals, particularly Calcium, Sodium and Phosphorus. The eyes need the whole gamut of these vitamins and minerals for good health.

One Japanese researcher Dr. Jin Otsuka, while denouncing sugar, goes to the extent of saying, ' if you give sugar to a rabbit, it will become myopic'. He relates the rise and fall of the incidence of myopia in Japan before and after World war II with the rise and fall of the supply of various refined foods, especially sugar. The more sugar in the diet, the greater the incidence of myopia. During the war years, the Japanese reverted to their traditional rise and fish diet, and prevalence of myopia plunged.

In conclusion, it can be said that vitamins, minerals and protein are extremely important for good eyes and good vision. Though each vitamin or mineral has its individual importance, it works better in conjunction with other vitamins. Teamwork is the key.

And it appears that a high intake of refined sugar makes their job difficult, since it burns up vitamins and minerals while it is being processed in the body.

It does not mean that supernutrition will enable you to throw away your glasses. But it does appear that it can be extremely beneficial in warding off and in some cases, actually healing-eye ailments.

We know that many persons will remain unconvinced about the significance of vitamins and minerals. 'My grandfather lived to be a hundred and he did not have much of vitamins'. But your grandfather probably did not live in a smog-saturated city, work under bright fluorescent lights or watch television. It is possible that your grandfather did not go to college nor was he anxious about scoring high marks – factors which overload our eyes with stress. Certainly, he did not eat convenient 'fast' foods, with much of their nutrients processed out and the flavour restored with additives. In other words, their vitamin and mineral requirements were minimal.

If the reader is genuinely interested in maintaining or improving the health of his body in general and his eyes in particular, he should analyse his diet and ensure an adequate supply of all the necessary nutrients.

References :

1. Borsook, Henry : Vitamins, What are they and how they can benefit you, The Viking Press, New York, 1940.

2. Clark, Linda : Get well naturally, Arco Press, New York, 1974.

3. Davis, Adelle : Let's eat right to keep fit, Harcourt Brace Jovanovich, New York, 1965.

4. Kirschmann, John D. : Nutrition Almanac, McGraw Hill, New York, 1975.

5. Rodale, J. : The Complete Book of Vitamins, Rodale Press, Emmaus, Pensylvania, 1977.

6. Rodale, J. : The Natural Way to Better Eyesight, Pyramid Books, New York, 1968.

7. Rosenberg, Harold and Fedlzamen : The Doctor's Book of Vitamin Therapy, G. P. Putnam's Sons, New York, 1974.

14. MAGNET THERAPY AND ACUPRESSURE

Magnet therapy is a comparatively new mode of treatment, which uses therapeutic magnets to influence various organs and body-processes suitably.

It has been observed or claimed by a number of researchers of international repute (and it is author's experience too) that the treatment of eyes with appropriate, weak magnets for about 15 to 30 minutes every day helps to preserve or improve eyesight and prevent eye-disorders.

In the treatment of eyes, the cooling and degeneration-retarding waves of the south-seeking (or simply south) pole of a magnet are utilised.

The south pole of a magnet, when placed adjacent to (or in contact with) an eye, produces the following effects :

(1) It relieves eye-strain and eye-pain by virtue of its cooling properties and thus refreshes the eye. This effect is useful in the prevention and control of visual errors and muscle-imbalances.

(2) It inhibits the activity of various micro-organisms (mainly bacteria) that may have happened to enter the eye.

This effect is useful in the prevention and control of eye-infections, especially those of the conjunctiva.

(3) It slows down degenerative processes occurring in the eye. This effect is useful in preventing or delaying eye-disorders of old age, like cataract.

It should be noted that the magnetic treatment of eyes is absolutely safe and entirely devoid of undesirable side-effects.

Acupressure is an ancient, oriental mode of treatment in which specific points on the surface of the body (i.e., the skin) are pressed to influence related internal organs of the body.

Acupressure is quite popular round the world, is an official mode of treatment in Oriental countries and has been recognised by the World Health Organisation (W.H.O.) as an authentic therapy.

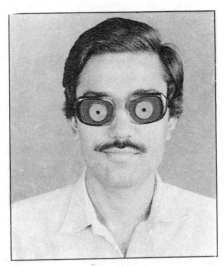

Fig. 14.1

How Acupressure works is still an unresolved mystery; but theories of neuro-humoral mechanisms have been propounded by researchers.

In China, noted for its studious and scholarly population, Acupressure is being extensively used to control myopia, a natural consequence of prolonged and unrelenting near-point work.

A number of Chinese researchers have claimed a reduction of upto one diopter of myopia, by treating the victims with Acupressure alone. However, the authors have found the effects of Acupressure to be less dramatic. Nevertheless, regular Acupressure can definitely control existent visual defects and associated symptoms like eye-strain, watering and headaches.

Acupressure points useful in the treatment and the control of visual defects have been depicted below :

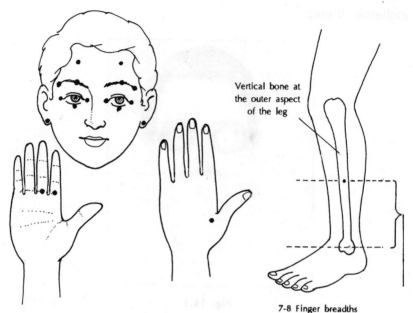

Vertical bone at the outer aspect of the leg

7-8 Finger breadths

Fig. 14.2

Each of the above points should be firmly and rythmically pressed with the tip of a finger (or the thumb) for about a minute, once or twice a day. Circular massage on the margin of orbital cavities (protective bony sockets in which the eye-balls are lodged) is also helpful.

In conclusion, it can be said that Magnet Therapy as well as Acupressure should also be employed with other modes of treatment like vision-training exercises and re-education of eye-use to prevent, control or diminish visual defects and eye-disorders.

15. FUTURE SIGHT : CARE OF CHILDREN'S EYES RIGHT FROM CHILDHOOD

Once upon a time, it was believed that heredity made a man. By this logic, intelligent, thrifty, loyal and wise parents would always produce children who were intelligent, thrifty, loyal and wise. It was in the genes. Conversely, children of a beggar or a thief did not stand much of a chance to be other than outcasts like their parents.

However, it did not always work out that way. History gives testimony to this fact. Dhondo Keshav Karve was born of very poor and illiterate parents. He pursued his entire education, reading and writing under street lights, yet he grew to become a great educationist and founded the S.N.D.T. University. Abraham Lincoln was born in a family of shepherds. Hitler's father painted people's homes. Charles Dicken's father was something of a scoundrel. Thomas Alva Edison's childhood was spent in utter poverty. Yet in later years, this genius of a scientist amassed fortune worth millions.

Present-day psychologists claim that a child is more or less a blank slate upon which certain behavioural patterns could be inscribed through conditioning. Environment affects not only the nature, the behaviour and the personality of a child but also its eyes and vision.

There are two ways to raise a child. We can let it grow and develop as chance and disposition dictate, basing parental guidance on intuition and the rules and rituals of the generation.

Or we can provide the child with an intellectually stimulating environment and coax and encourage the youngster to develop intelligence in order to achieve success in our world, to be a doctor, an engineer or a chartered accountant. But we may do so at the expense of the child's vision.

When a child walks through school doors for the first time, it enters the adult visual world where it will be assaulted with a complex network of tiny details–letters and numbers – through which it is expected to learn. On the first day of school, its life is altered drastically from one of days of fun and games to long periods of sitting still and concentrating.

The educational system seems designed to ruin its sight by requiring it to attend to details hour after hour and the result can be seen in the fact that roughly half of the population wear glasses. Obviously, this is not a call to shut down schools but an attempt to make parents and educators think about what we are doing, albeit inadvertently, in our traditional halls of learning : causing visual havoc.

If schools cannot be closed down, what is the other way out ? It is simply this : make the eyes capable of withstanding the onslaught by taking correct steps and ensuring that the eyes develop into strong appendages. This requires that parents help a child learn how to use its eyes properly, how to see properly. We hold a toddler's hand when it takes its first shaky steps while learning to walk; its eyes need a different kind of help. Because we can't see a pair of eyes grow up and learn doesn't mean that they don't do so.

The amount of research regarding how eyes grow and vision develops has accumulated to the point where we can no longer afford to be unaware of what is going on in a child's eye and blithely assume that everything will turn out for the best.

How a child grows and learns and is able to use its eyes which are the windows to the world, will largely determine its abilities to carry itself on through life. Although all the skills– motor, sensory and mental–play their individual part in a whole person, the visual abilities are primarily responsible for co-ordinating the system. For the twentieth century man, vision is especially critical since so much of the information he gains about the world comes to him through his eyes. In our literate culture, we ask eyes to take on a job for which evolution has not yet prepared them : close concentration hour after hour, paying attention to details, reading words, adding or substracting numbers or operating a computer. The message of the time is clear : succeed and achieve in this manner or fall by the wayside. No wonder, visual problems are on the rise.

But there is a great deal a parent can do to help a child develop strong eyes, healthy vision and adult perception. The development of the eyes starts right at conception and continues after the child is born and attains an age of six years. If the child's eyes are to be given a fighting chance against the visual requirements of life today, intelligent care is essential. The various stages in the development of the eyes and the vision and steps to be taken have been described below :

Birth to two months : That the eyes commence their movements even before birth has been determined by specific instruments.

At birth, a child is able to move its eyes momentarily, but usually one at a time. It looks at you now with one eye and then with the other. Its focusing ability is limited to a few inches from its face. Seeing clearly those objects which are more than 7-8 inches away from the eyes is not possible.

At this stage, eye movements are closely linked to body movement : when it looks, it stops moving and when it moves, it stops looking !

Even in the first week, the infant has some basic survival instincts incorporated into its visual mechanism. It will try to avoid an object approaching its face.

In the second week, the child will be attracted to sounds and lights and will attempt to turn its eyes towards them. At night, it has something to look at.

The cradle in which the child sleeps should have open or transparent sides which would allow it to see through. At this age, the child is not able to move its head on its own. Hence, do not keep the cradle near a wall. Otherwise, the child will not receive stimulation to use both its eyes. If the cradle has to be kept near a wall, the child's position should be frequently changed so that light coming from various directions enters and stimulates its eyes.

By the time the child is five to six weeks old, it is aware of different patterns. Hang a toy on its cradle, about a foot from its eyes. Talk to it from different areas of the room. This gives it a chance to watch and follow a moving target and allows it to associate distance and direction with both sight and hearing.

Let your child spend some of its waking time in rooms other than its nursery. Providing it with more bright areas and objects to watch while it is learning to control it eye-movements.

Encourage the child to move its head by placing it on its stomach for five to ten minutes at a time.

Two to four months : Somewhere around fourteen weeks, the eyes begin to converge, enabling the child to judge the distance of various objects from it, i.e., to determine which object is closer than the other.

The child also tries to reach nearby objects with its arms and legs, developing the co-ordination between eyes and limbs in the process.

Continue to place the child on its stomach for short periods of time so that its ability to move its head develops further.

Toys and other things to reach should still be within eight inches, the distance it can focus.

Four to six months : The child now is able to turn itself from one side to the other and its use of arms and legs is picking up. Thus eye-hand co-ordination develops further.

Make sure that the child can look out of the cradle on both sides and has interesting things to look at.

Six to eight months : By the sixth month, the child can use both its eyes together and in co-ordination.

Simple games can prove useful in developing its visual abilities. Play hide and seek games. Put a ball under a blanket and ask it to locate it. Roll a ball back and forth to it. Make it sit so that the ball will roll between its legs. This will develop the ability of its eyes to track moving objects. Provide it with stacking toys, stuffed animals and objects with details. The child is ready to look at finer points of larger objects.

Eight to fourteen months : The child now uses its eyes to judge distance and throw objects with precision.

Provide it with simple toys, the parts of which can be taken apart and then assembled together. Also continue to give it objects which roll, such as balls.

Fourteen months to two years : The child should have its depth perception fairly well developed and its body co-ordinated at this stage, so that walking, going up and down steps on four limbs, jumping and running are accomplished easily. Eye-hand co-ordination is fairly smooth.

Two to three years : This is a good time to make the child aware of good visual habits.

Prevent the child from taking undue interest in near-point activities. Insist that the child does all reading, writing or drawing in sitting posture only, in very good light and keeping a fair distance between its eyes and the book. Continuously instruct child in this regard.

Habits like this are not formed overnight, which is why adults reading this book and having best intentions of following our suggestions, often have difficulty remembering to do them !

Three to five years : The suggestions for children from two to three years, apply to a greater extent at this stage.

The child's activities should be balanced. It should not be sedentary all the time, nor should it always be outdoors running and jumping. It will have too much trouble when school starts. But the little girl who has learned how to read and does not want to do anything else or the youngster who has three to four hours of television or video viewing daily needs to be encouraged to use her / his muscles and move her / his body through space. In short, see to it that your child grows up into a flexible adult with more than one way of expressing himself or herself.

The child should also be taught the ways of cleaning and resting the eyes. It should also be taught to let its body-muscles go limp and slack, through Shavasana.

Get your child's eyes and sight examined before admitting it to a school. Such eye check-ups should be repeated every six months thereafter.

If your child is clumsy, if it trips or falls over objects or bumps into them, if it just cannot concentrate on reading, colouring or drawing, if it thrusts its head forward to look at distant objects, if its eyes do not seem straight, if it blinks more often or shuts its eyes partially while viewing television, if it tilts its head to one side, if it holds the book too close to its eyes or if it complains of headaches, dizziness and watering from the eyes after spending time on a visual task, it could be having a visual shortcoming or defect. An early detection and prompt treatment may bring an end to the problem.

If one of the two parents (or both) have visual defects, they should be all the more alert and prevent such a development in their children.

16. CONTACT LENSES

During the past few years, the demand for and the use of contact lenses have shown an unprecedented increase. It is necessary to enlighten people about some facts and fallacies regarding contact lenses.

The first contact lens came into existence in 1887. This lens was double-walled and was made of glass. The lens contained between its two walls, a substance called gelatin. At that time, however, there was no way of measuring the anterior curvature of the eye-ball. Hence the lens did not fit well on the eye and had to be discarded. In 1932, Dr. Joseph Dallos succeeded in measuring the curvature of the eye-ball and prepared a glass contact lens accordingly. This lens, however, happened to be too heavy to be worn comfortably even for a few seconds. In 1943, plastic contact lenses made their appearance. These lenses were made to fit on whole of the outer surface of the eye-ball and were termed scleral contact lenses. In 1948, corneal contact lenses came into existence. Such lenses are fitted only on the transparent part of the eye, i.e., cornea.

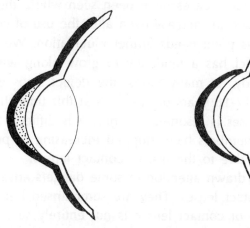

Fig. 16.1 : Scleral contact lens   **Fig. 16.2 : Corneal contact lens**
This lens is now obsolete.   This lens is widely used nowadays.

At present three types of corneal contact lenses are available : hard, semisoft and soft. Each has its own advantages and disadvantages.

There are a few eye-defects which are more amenable to contact lenses than to glasses. Contact lenses are of great value in correcting high astigmatism (irregular sight), keratoconus (cone-shaped cornea) and high anisometropia (big difference in refractory powers of the two eyes). Correction of high anisometropia with glasses usually results into double vision. This difficulty can be overcome with contact lenses.

Certain defects arising out of the use of glasses can be overcome with contact lenses. A person can see clearly only if he sees through the centre of the glass. Peripheral or paracentral parts of glasses give rise to defects like spherical aberration, chromatic aberration and coma. Due to this, the person has to contend with a limited field of vision. On the other hand, since the contact lenses move with the eyes, one always sees through the centres of the lenses. Hence the question of above mentioned defects does not arise.

It is said that contact lenses help to check the increase of eye-defect and the number (of spectacles) becomes steady. However, innumerable cases have been seen where the eye-defect has continued to increase even after the use of contact lenses. In fact, this point needs further elucidation. We know that a visual defect has a tendency to grow along with the growth of the body. In many cases, the defect stops getting worse at around 17-18 years of age. It is at this time that the use of contact lenses is resorted to. Thus, it is difficult to say whether the eye-numbers have stopped increasing as per the natural course or due to the use of contact lenses.

Experts have drawn attention to some dangers arising out of the use of contact lenses. They are summarised below :

(1) The use of contact lenses is not entirely safe.

(2) If strict hygienic conditions are not maintained during insertion or removal of contact lenses, the eyes may get contaminated with germs and micro-organisms.

(3) The cornea solely depends upon atmospheric oxygen for its nutrition. Contact lenses do not allow atmospheric oxygen to come in contact with cornea. This results into corneal oedema (water-logging).

(4) If proper care is not taken while inserting or removing a contact lens, the cornea might be injured resulting into abrasions and scratches which affect vision.

Thus ophthalmologists have thrown light on probable dangers of contact lenses' use. Though such complications are rare, one should be aware of them.

The dangers of contact lenses' use mostly arise if the contact lenses do not fit properly on the eyes. If the lens is prepared without precisely measuring the anterior curvature of the cornea, a number of difficulties like redness and pain in the eyes, corneal sweeling, corneal abrasions, decrease in corneal transparency etc. arise. However, these difficulties do not arise if the lenses are of precise shape, i.e., if their fitting is proper.

A person who opts for contact lenses initially experiences certain difficulties. His eyes water continuously, he experiences dust in his eyes and the rate of blinking increases. Excessive tears sometimes cause displacement of the lens resulting into a red-eye. In some persons, difficulties last about one to four weeks. But if lenses are properly fitted, such difficulties shortly disappear. The extent of such difficulties is much lesser with soft or semisoft lenses.

In conclusion, it can be said that use of contact lenses has its own advantages and disadvantages. However, if the lenses are prepared by an expert and if they are properly fitted, the incidence of difficulties is negligible.

The advantages of their use are obvious. Appearance improves; question of distortion of objects arising out of vision through peripheral parts of glasses does not arise; objects appear to be of their normal size (not larger or smaller as happens with glasses) In some cases, the visual defect stops increasing.

The reader should opt for contact lenses only after giving thought to all aspects of their advantages and disadvantages.

---

17. THE OPERATION TO REDUCE EYE-NUMBERS : RADIAL KERATOTOMY

People off and on seek advice regarding the surgery for bringing down the eye-numbers.

People desire to be able to see clearly without glasses. Such a desire is natural. To satisfy such desire, four different types of operations have been tried : (1) Radial keratotomy (2) Keratophakia (3) Epikeratophakia and (4) Keratomileusis.

Of these, the later three operations are too complicated to perform and have given inconsistent results. Hence they have not become popular with surgeons. The first operation–radial keratotomy has gained considerable popularity.

In 1939, Dr. Sutomu Sato of Japan first thought of this operation. However, the results of the operations he performed were disastrous.

Thereafter in 1969, Dr. Yanaliev of Russia gave a new lease of life to this operation. He performed this operation on 500 persons and achieved a success rate of about 70%.

In 1972, Dr. Fyodorov of Russia performed 5000 such operations with great success. Dr. Fyodorov became instrumental in spreading the popularity of this operation in many countries of the world.

What is actually done in this operation ?

In a way, the operation is quite simple. It is usually performed on persons suffering from short sight. The operation consists of making 8 to 16 radial incisions on the cornea.

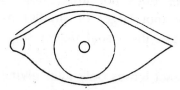 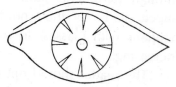

Fig. 17.1 : Normal cornea　　Fig. 17.2 : Cornea after operation

This results into flattening of the cornea. Parallel rays of light, which previously converged to a focus in front of the retina, now come to a focus exactly on the retina and the person sees clearly.

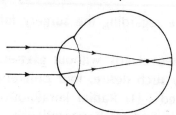 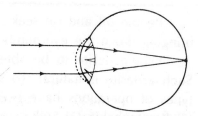

Fig. 17.3 : Before operation
In myopia, parallel rays of light come to a focus in front of the retina.

Fig. 17.4 : After operation
The cornea has been flattened so that parallel rays of light get focussed on the retina.

The diagrams above depict the ideal results of the operation. However, such ideal results are obtained only in a few cases, the details of which have been discussed later in this chapter.

Who can undergo this operation ?

(1) A person who is free of any eye-disease.

(2) A person who is atleast 17-18 years old.

(3) A person whose eye-numbers have stabilised.

The last point needs further elucidation. It is clear that if the visual defect is of a progressive nature, the operation is usually not undertaken. This is due to the fact that this operation can bring down numbers, but it cannot stop them from increasing.

Some experts claim a reduction of 5-6 diopters in eye-numbers after this surgery. But the observed fact is that, on an average, the operation brings down the number by 1.5 to 2.5 diopters. A person using glasses of power greater than 2.5 diopters and desirous of completely doing away with glasses may have to undergo this operation twice or thrice, at intervals of a few days. However, many eye-surgeons strongly advise against a second operation on the same eye.

As stated earlier, during the operation, the cornea is incised at 8 to 16 places. The determination of the exact depth of incisions entails complicated calculations. Even after laborious calculations, it might not be possible to make incisions of the desired depth. The most important thing is that, after the operation, the process and rate of healing differs from person to person. The eye-number, therefore, does not get reduced by the desired extent. Thus, the eye-numbers can rarely be brought down to zero. In other words, even after the operation, a person has to use glasses (possibly of lesser powers). In short, the desire of discarding glasses is seldom fulfilled.

Dr. Ranga Reddy and his colleagues performed such 140 operations at the Sarojinidevi Eye Hospital in Hyderabad. Thereafter, for five years, the persons were continuously kept under observation. The report of unaided visual acuity (i.e., sight without glasses) of these 140 persons has been given below :

Observation No.	Visual Acuity	No. of patients	Percentage
1	6/6	none	–
2	6/9	none	–
3	6/12	9	6.5%
4	6/18	21	15.0%
5	6/24	52	37.5%
6	6/60 or less	58	41.0%
		140	100.0%

The above table shows that only 21.5% of all patients obtained useful unaided sight (6/12 or 6/18) after the operation. None of the patients could obtain really sharp vision.

Dangers and complications of R. K. operation :

(1) The extent of decrease in eye-numbers cannot even be roughly predicted.

(2) For a period of one to six months following the operation, the vision continues to fluctuate. Till the vision stabilises, new glasses cannot be prescribed.

(3) In many cases within 3 to 5 years, the visual defect returns with a vengeance. This is the experience of Dr. Ranga Reddy. The long-term report of 140 such operations performed at the Sarojinidevi Eye Hospital has been given below :

Observation No.	Change in eye-numbers after the operation	No. of Patients	Percentage
1	A decrease of 2 diopters	12	9%
2	A decrease of 1 diopter	44	31%
3	No decrease at all, i.e., nos. increased to the original level	84	60%

Dr. Ranga Reddy bluntly states that any reduction in eye-numbers obtained immediately after the operation is apparent and temporary. The table given above is a testimony to this fact.

(4) Persons who undergo this operation show a decreased tolerance to light. According to Dr. Casimir Swinger, an eminent ophthalmologist associated with America's Mount Sinai School of Medicine and Beth Israel Medical Centre, 50 to 79 % of all persons continue to suffer from photophobia and glare even six months after the operation.

(5) If the corneal incision turns out to be deeper than desired, the cornea may get perforated with disastrous results. Complications that occur include injury and inflammation of the iris, injury to the eye-lens, endopthalmitis (inflammation of all eye-tissues) and formation of cataract.

(6) After the operation, in many cases, the corneal surface becomes irregular and uneven. In such cases, normal sight cannot be restored with glasses or contact lenses.

(7) Pus-forming organisms might grow in the corneal incisions. In severe cases, corneal ulcers might result and sight may be lost.

(8) An important fact that should be considered is that this operation only alters the shape of the cornea and thereby brings down eye-numbers. It does nothing to strengthen the weak tissues of the eyes. Degenerative changes of the retina and vitreous that are associated with high myopia (short-sightedness) continue to progress.

In conclusion, it can be said that the operation carries with it, too many risks. With glasses most of the persons come to possess good sight. After the eye-numbers become steady, this sight lasts for the whole life. Then why should anybody go for an operation which might endanger the sight or the eye ? It should also be remembered that short-sightedness is only a defect of the eye and not a disease. Any operation, however simple, has its own inherent complications.

It is possible that with advance of technique and with invention of better instruments, the operation will become safer in years to come. But considering the present circumstances, it would not be an exaggeration to say that at present, doing appropriate eye-exercises or using contact lenses is a better solution to the problem of near-sightedness than opting for an operation for reducing eye-numbers.

18. A BACKLOG OF ESSENTIAL QUESTIONS & ANSWERS

Q. 1. My vision has diminished gradually. I cannot see distant objects clearly. Will vision-training restore my vision ?

Ans. A gradual diminution in vision might be due to a functional cause (i.e., due to a refractive error like myopia or due to amblyopia) or due to a pathological cause (like cataract).

Vision-training can act to overcome functional diminution of vision, that is to say it can control or improve a refractive error. But, as is obvious, it can have no effect upon a pathological condition of the eye.

Only an eye-specialist can accurately diagnose the cause for diminution of vision. However, even a layman can guess the cause with as simple a device as a small disc having a pin-hole. If, on seeing through the pinhole, the vision seems to improve considerably, the diminution of vision may be safely considered to be due to a refractive error. On the other hand, if the vision does not improve on seeing through the pin-hole, the impairment of vision cannot be attributed to a refractive error and an eye-disease is likely to be present, calling for a visit to an eye-doctor.

Q. 2. Which, apart from cataract, are the pathological causes for gradual diminution of vision ?

Ans. The commonest pathological causes for gradual diminution of vision are :

(1) **Cataract,** which is a condition in which the crystalline lens present inside the eye loses its transparency.

(2) **Simple chronic glaucoma,** which is a sinister condition in which the pressure of the fluids inside the eye-ball (called intra-ocular tension) remains elevated, gradually damaging the cells and tissues of the eye.

(3) **Diabetic retinopathy,** which is a degenerative condition of the retina, brought about by longstanding diabetes.

(4) **Hypertensive retinopathy,** which is a degenerative condition of the retina, brought about by longstanding high blood pressure.

(5) **Toxic amblyopia,** which is a degenerative condition of the retina and the optic nerve brought about by long term use of intoxicants like alcohol, tobacco etc.

All these conditions call for treatment by an eye-doctor.

Surgery provides a satisfactory solution to the problem of cataract.

Toxic amblyopia improves if the victim abstains from the causative intoxicant and is given vitamins in large doses.

The remaining three causes for diminution of vision do not satisfactorily respond, even to the best treatment. Treatment can, however, prevent further worsening of the condition.

Thus, all these are grave pathological conditions which do not fall into the province of vision therapy.

Q. 3. Can elders, too, undertake vision-training to improve their eye-sight and strengthen their eyes ?

Ans. For undertaking vision-training, there is no age-bar. However, the fact remains that in old persons, the various tissues of the eyes are not as flexible or malleable as those in the young. Hence, improvement in old persons may be slow or even turn out be incomplete.

Q. 4. I have crossed eyes. Will vision-training help to straighten my eyes ?

Ans. There are various types of squint. Some types of squint are amenable to vision therapy exercises and other non-invasive measures.

In other types of squint, vision therapy exercises do not give consistent results. However, every person suffering from squint should give vision therapy a fair try, before considering surgery.

It should be noted that the results of surgery for squint are often unsatisfactory; that is to say, surgery more often than not fails to completely straighten the eye. Even when the eyes do become straight following surgery, they should be constantly exercised using the principles of vision therapy, to prevent a recurrence of the squint.

Simultaneous binocular vision and fusion are the primary requisites for straight eyes. Unless these are subsequently developed and maintained, surgery is likely to turn out a failure in the long run.

Q. 5. Can vision-training exercise help an aphakic (a person who has undergone cataract surgery) ?

Ans. The crystalline lens inside our eye is normally transparent. When it turns opaque, the victim is said to be suffering from cataract. An opaque lens prevents light rays from reaching the retina, thereby diminishing the vision. In cataract surgery, this opaque lens, which obstructs the light rays, is removed.

As stated earlier, the various tissues and coats of an elderly person's eyes are not flexible enough to allow an actual reduction in eye-numbers.

However, vision-training exercises can definitely make an aphakic person's eyes and muscles more efficient and strong, thereby enhancing the quality of his or her vision.

Q. 6. Can vision-training help night-blindness or colour blindness ?

Ans. Night-blindness is a condition in which the vision is defective at night but good in the day-time. It may be due to :

(1) Hereditary causes

(2) Retinal causes (e.g., retinitis pigmentosa)

(3) Systemic causes (e.g., vitamin A deficiency)

Colour-blindness is a condition in which the victim has defective colour discrimination. It may be congenital (hereditary) or acquired (following a disease of the retina or the optic nerve).

A congenital defect cannot be cured or helped by any form of treatment. Night or colour blindness due to retinal or systemic causes sometimes improves with appropriate medical or nutritional treatment.

Obviously, vision therapy has no role to play in the treatment of night-blindness or colour-blindness.

Q. 7. Can vision-training exercises help nystagmus ?

Ans. Nystagmus is a condition characterised by involuntary and continuous to and fro movements of the eyes. It is usually bilateral (i.e., affects both eyes equally) and regular. The movements of the eyes may be horizontal, vertical or tortional in nature.

The shakiness of the eyes in nystagmus becomes accentuated when looking to either side (i.e., when not looking straight ahead). Sometimes it appears only when one eye is covered (latent nystagmus).

Nystagmus may be ocular (i.e., due to eye causes), labyrinthine (i.e., due to some defect of the labyrinth of the ear) or central (i.e., due to some damage to the cerebellum or brain-stem).

More often than not, nystagmus is found associated with some defect of vision (refractive error). As a result of the unsteadiness of the eyes and the simultaneous presence of a visual defect, the victim's vision is quite poor.

Vision-training can have no direct effect on nystagmus. However, it may help to control the associated visual error and thereby improve vision.

Q. 8. How frequently should the vision and eyes be tested ?

Ans. The eyes of a child should be examined before it enters a school. If nothing is found wrong or if the child has no complaints, its eye may be tested every six months or every year thereafter. However, if the child's eyes and vision are found to be lacking in some respect during the first examination, it becomes necessary that repeat examinations be carried out every three months.

The results of such tests should be recorded on a special card, a model of which has been depicted below :

Date	
Vision without ⟨ R glasses ⟨ L	- - - - - - - - - - - - - - -
Vision with glasses ⟨ R (indicate the ⟨ L power)	- - - - - - - - - - - - - - -

Such a chart becomes a source of ready reference and indicates whether the visual defect is progressive or stationary.

Elders, too, should get their eyes examined at yearly intervals.

Parents having visual defects should remain alert and get their child's eyes examined more frequently than usual because such children have greater chances of developing similar visual defects.

Q. 9. Will vision-training enable me to discard my glasses ?

Ans. We possess 'stone-age' eyes, that is to say that their evolution has not kept pace with the rest of our body. In other words, our eyes are not strong enough to fulfil the heavy visual demands which we thrust upon them. Hence they break down. It is no wonder that visual defects are on the rise. The unsurpassable demands which our educational system places upon the tender eyes of small children is the reason why we see even tiny tots sporting glasses.

Vision-training seeks to render the eyes strong yet flexible, so as to enable them to withstand the onslaught they are subjected to. This goal is achieved by a process consisting of specific eye-exercises and visual re-education.

It is possible that this process may act to enable some persons to discontinue the use of glasses (and indeed, you may have bought this book with that goal in mind). But in its total extent, vision therapy's goals are far more superior. It strives to make the eyes stronger and vision more flexible so that the person is able to cope with the present-day visual demands with ease and confidence, without harming his or her eyes.

Q. 10. As my vision improves, will I have to go on changing my glasses or contact lenses ?

Ans. To see clearly through a particular pair of glasses, the eyes have to constantly maintain that much defect, which the glasses are made to correct.

Therefore, it is desirable that after the eye-number comes down by a substantial amount, the glasses be changed.

If a person continues to wear glasses stronger than he or she actually requires, his or her sight may not improve further or the eye-numbers may shoot up again.

The curvature and the power of hard or semi-soft contact lenses can be changed to a certain extent by regrinding them. This procedure does not entail much expenditure.

Q. 11. What are symptoms that may indicate vision problems in a child ?

Ans. A child, which is old enough to converse, will usually complain of difficulty in seeing.

However, in all children the following symptoms should arouse a suspicion of a visual problem :

(1) Rubbing the eyes

(2) Closing or covering one eye

(3) Squinting while looking at the blackboard

(4) Partial shutting of the eyes when looking at the T.V. set or other distant objects

(5) Insistence on viewing the T.V. set from a close range

(6) Holding reading material very close to the eyes

(7) Headaches after reading or writing

(8) Tilting the head to one side

(9) Confusing similar words

(10) A disinclination for close range works like reading, writing, drawing and painting.

(11) Persistent letter or word reversal

(12) Frequently overlooking or missing letters or misspeling words while copying from the blackboard

(13) Drop in school grades as the child advances to higher standards

(14) Blurring of vision at any time.

Besides, if a child displays an excessive leaning towards a particular visual style (see chapter 16), it might be suffering from a visual defect or has the likelihood of developing one in the future.

If a child exhibits one of the many symptoms enlisted above, it should be taken to a eye-specialist without delay. The importance of catching and treating a visual defect as early as possible (i.e., nipping a defect in its bud) cannot be overemphasized.

Q. 12. Can a eye-defect or a visual defect give rise to headaches ?

Ans. An eye-strain due to an ocular or a visual defect may be the cause of headache. It should, however, be understood that the relationship between headache and a visual defect has been overemphasized (blown out of proportion).

Headache is more often a result of other disorders like mental tension or sinus problems. In fact, there are about twenty-five causes of headache, with visual defects occupying a place at the bottom of the list.

A headache arising due to a visual defect is never severe and can more accurately be described as a heaviness of the head. It is located in the forehead just above the eye-brows and occurs only after the eyes have been employed in some work requiring intense concentration. Such headache is quickly relieved if the eyes are rested.

Therefore, when you next suffer from a headache, don't go rushing to a eye-doctor !

Q. 13. I have heard of a special method of reducing eye-numbers by using contact lenses. What is it ?

Ans. The system is called orthokeratology and it is usually employed for myopics. In myopia, the cornea is more curved than normal. In orthokeratology, progressively flatter contact lenses are fitted on the eyes with a view to somewhat flattening the cornea, thereby reducing the eye numbers.

Even if one were to accept that orthokeratology does bring down eye-numbers, two points should be well understood :

(1) Flat contact lenses can never be comfortable.

(2) Even after bringing down the numbers to the desired level, a person has to continue wearing contact lenses to maintain the improvement. If the use of contact lenses is discontinued, the cornea usually reverts back to its original shape (i.e., regains its original curvature), thereby bringing back the eye-numbers.

Besides, the cost of undergoing this treatment is quite prohibitive.

Q. 14. Can an aphakic person (one who has undergone cataract surgery) wear contact lenses ?

Ans. In cataract surgery, the crystalline lens inside the eye is removed. To compensate for this removed lens, an aphakic will have to wear either glasses or contact lenses.

Since glasses remain at some distance from the eyes, they tend to alter the size of the viewed objects. Greater the power of the glasses, the greater is the magnification or minification (as the case may be) of the viewed object.

An aphakic usually requires convex lens of +10 to +12 diopters (numbers). If he opts for glasses, he sees objects twenty per cent larger than they actually are. If only one eye has been operated for cataract, this twenty per cent difference in the size of images formed in the two eyes causes great problems. The brain cannot fuse such dissimilar images, resulting into double vision.

Contact lenses provide an answer to this problem. Since contact lenses remain in contact with the eyes, they do not cause an alteration (i.e., magnification or diminution) in the size of the viewed object.

Another point of importance is that a glass provides clear vision only if one sees through its centre. Vision gets distorted if one were to see through peripheral parts of a glass. Thus an aphakic is forced to move his head (instead of his eyes) every time he wishes to change his view. On the other hand, since contact lenses move along with the eyes, one always sees through their optical centres, no matter whether he sees straight ahead or in any other direction.

Q. 15. Are there any norms to be followed while selecting the shape of the frame or the type of glasses ?

Ans. Frame : (1) If your visual defect is large (i.e., if you have been prescribed a high power), choose a small frame so that the glasses can be kept reasonably thin. Big glasses (that would fit in a big frame) are not only heavier but also give rise to distorted vision when you see through their peripheral parts.

(2) Ensure that your eyes come to lie behind the geometrical centres of the frame apertures; otherwise your vision will not only be hazy but distorted too.

Unless the optical centres of the lenses and the eyes coincide, vision cannot be good or comfortable even if the frame looks good on your face or the glasses have been made accurately as per the doctor's prescription. Indeed, such a person then shuttles between the doctor (who reiterates that the prescription is correct) and the optician (who is adamant that the glasses are correct).

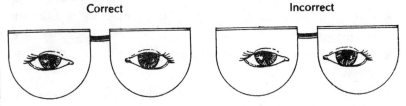

Correct	Incorrect
Central position of eyes behind glasses	Eccentric position of eyes behind glasses

Glasses : Generally speaking, white (or colourless) glasses are best for the eyes since they allow all seven colours of the spectrum to enter the eyes.

Never opt for tinted glasses unless your eyes are extremely sensitive to light. In fact, a better solution to photophobia (abnormal sensitivity to light) is to desensitize the eyes by exposing them to sun for progressively greater lengths of time, taking care never to look directly at the sun. With such treatment, the photophobia quickly disappears.

The so called 'day and night' or automatic (photochromatic) glasses, which change their colour according to the intensity of light, should also be avoided. Our eyes have an in-built mechanism (effected by the muscles of the iris) to control the amount of light entering the eyes. Our pupils become small in bright light and expand in dim light ! Wearing photo-chromatic glasses gradually weakens the muscles of the iris.

Published by Navneet Publications (India) Ltd., Dantali, Gujarat.
Printed by   Tri : Shaktiya Print & Book Finishin, Ahd. – 380 004.

AUTO-URINE THERAPY

If we can drink the urine of cows, why can't we drink our own urine?

Free your mind of the misguided disgust about urine and regain your lost health.

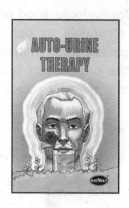

- Has your illness resisted all kinds of treatment?
- Are there no specific medicines for your illness?
- Are you apprehensive about the side-effects of drugs?
- Have you despaired of life?

DO NOT LOSE HOPE.

HAVE RECOURSE TO AUTO-URINE THERAPY.

Our ancient Vedic works too, have recommended the drinking of one's own urine. In the Damar Tantra, composed by Lord Shiva Himself, auto-urine has been described as 'Shivambu', 'Shiva' means 'salubrious or beneficial, and 'ambu' means 'water'. Thus the combined term, 'shivambu' means salubrious water.

- A large number of supposedly incurable diseases have been successfully treated with self-urine. Cases of complete cure of even a disease like cancer have been recorded.
- The idea that urine is nothing but a poisonous waste rejected by the body is a total misconception.
- Barring exceptional cases, fresh urine is always completely free from micro-organisms (bacteria) of all kinds.
- Urine contains hormones, enzymes, vitamins and numerous other nutritive and curative substances.

A book containing a complete exposition of the scientific basis of AUTO-URINE THERAPY.

E 8